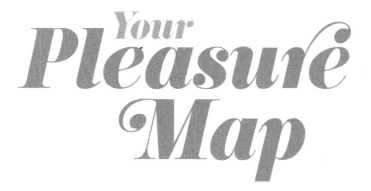

Your Pleasure Map

A WOMAN'S Q&A GUIDE
TO HOTTER, HEALTHIER, MORE
ADVENTUROUS SEX

Tina Katz, M.ED, ACS

Amorata
Press

Published by: Amorata Press
          an imprint of Ulysses Press
          PO Box 3440
          Berkeley, CA 94703
          www.ulyssespress.com

ISBN: 978-1-61243-275-5
Library of Congress Control Number: 2013914553

Printed in the United States
10 9 8 7 6 5 4 3 2 1

Acquisitions editor: Keith Riegert
Project editor: Katherine Furman
Managing editor: Claire Chun
Front cover design: Chalkley Calderwood
Cover photo: ©Nejron Photo/shutterstock.com
Interior design and layout: Wade Nights
Indexer: Jay Kreider, J S Editorial

Contents

Introduction

How to Use Your Pleasure Map

Hello.

There are countless ways that *Your Pleasure Map* could have ended up in your hands. Perhaps you're a self-assured and sassy woman, and the idea of getting to choose your own sexual adventures appealed to you. Perhaps you're more of a sexual newbie looking for some tips and techniques to help bring out your inner bedroom goddess. Whatever it was that made you pick up this book, rest assured that it's for you, because you're the one who decides how to make it work for you. You can use this book any way you want. Each chapter poses several scenarios and then gives you "pick your passion" options for different outcomes. *Your Pleasure Map* is designed so you can pick whatever turns you on the most and read all about it. You'll discover creative yet practical ways to go on new adventures tailor-made to your desires. With all the options explored between these covers, you're bound to find turn-ons that you never imagined before or that you just never really considered. You'll also get the scoop on how to make these fantasies part of your reality.

Even though this book is a map to lead you to new frontiers, you don't have to pick just one passion in each scenario. You may want to read this book from beginning to end, chapter after chapter, and glean from it everything you can. You may decide to read only those sections that interest you. You may find yourself reading the adventurous options aloud to your partner (or partners) and have fun and interesting conversations about how you each answered.

Why write a book for women on how to be sexually empowered? Why should there be something written specifically for women to examine their own sexuality, look at their body image, learn about anatomy, and give them ways to consider what makes them feel sexually confident?

Because of the way our society views sex, sexuality, and especially women, there aren't a lot of opportunities for women to get real information. While there are a plethora of periodical publications that you can pick up at the checkout stand of the grocery store or access online, they tend to simply state and restate the same few tips that focus almost solely on the man's pleasure (and they tend to be very heterocentric). If you're lucky, you might get some form of comprehensive sex education in middle school or high school. But following graduation, you're left to figure the rest out for yourself. Even many of the best comprehensive sexuality education programs don't include any information on pleasure and communication, and frequently don't even have the clitoris on the vaginal/vulvar anatomy pictures. The clitoris is a body part designed for nothing more than the sole purpose of providing pleasure (which is a pretty amazing feat in and of itself), and we as a society pretend it just flat out doesn't exist. Then, once you turn eighteen, or you graduate high school, magically you're now allowed to become a sexual being and are supposed to have exciting, fulfilling, and engaging sexual experiences, as well as authentic, communicative relationships. It's a wonderful concept and a fabulous thing to aim for, but how can we all hope to attain these goals when we've been given no education, no guidance, and no direction on how to make these sexually satisfying and emotionally fulfilling interactions happen?

I believe that making education about sexuality and relationships for all adults accessible is so important that I decided to become a board-certified sexologist and sex educator who works specifically with adults. This book came out of the idea that sexually empowering women to have the sex lives that they want is a radical idea that can support women of all relationship statuses, orientations, ages, economic statuses, ability levels, ethnic backgrounds, races, and more.

While every adult has the right to inclusive and accessible sex education, our society is determined to undermine women's sexuality. There's the Madonna/Whore complex: if you don't know enough about sex, you're mocked as being innocent and naive, but if you have information about sex and are willing to share it, discuss it, and use it, you're viewed as slutty, skanky, and easy.

Both of these options are unacceptable to me. Everyone should have a smorgasbord of information available to them about sexuality, and they can choose in each situation or scenario which bits and pieces they want to use. There shouldn't be any stigma about choosing not to be sexually active, just as there shouldn't be any stigma about possessing information on sexuality and choosing to explore and celebrate your sexuality. These binaries and stereotypes are used for nothing more than to control women and their bodies, and it needs to stop.

So read this book. Read it as part of a book club. Read it on the train (no, don't cover up the title). Read it while you're waiting for your kids to get out of practice. Read it at the gym. Read it on the plane. Read it in front of your partner. You should have the right to gain sexual confidence anywhere, anytime. We shouldn't be ashamed of wanting information about sex, sexuality, relationships, bodies, communication, and more. Everyone wants this info—heck, look how popular *Fifty Shades of Grey* was, across generations, regions, and other different demographics. Even my mother-in-law asked me about it. If women all over the world can get their jollies reading a book about men dominating women in the bedroom, then they should also be able to read a book about empowering women sexually so that they have the sex they want to have, when they want to have it!

The full title of this book is *Your Pleasure Map: A Woman's Q&A Guide to Hotter, Naughtier, More Adventurous Sex.* I have to tell you, I had some reservations about using the word *naughtier*. While the word has some appeal (I mean, seriously, who doesn't want to read a book that talks about naughty sex?!), I want us to move away from the common notion of naughty sex being sex that's anything other than penis-in-vagina, missionary-style sex, and that wanting to have fulfilling/interesting/creative sex is somehow a trait of "bad girls" and that "good girls" have to become naughty in some way to have sexually satisfying encounters. To that, I stick out my tongue (and do some licking with it).

Sex is never inherently good or bad, regardless of what sex acts you're discussing or whom you're doing them with. Good sex is sex that feels good, that fulfills your wants and needs, and makes you feel, well, good. Bad sex is sex that's done because it's what you're "supposed" to do: it's boring, unfulfilling, or may even feel bad.

Good girls can have good sex and bad sex, as can bad girls. And while we're at it, let's throw the whole concept of using the term *girls* to refer to adult women out the window. Of course, if being called a good girl or a bad girl helps get you off, I'm all for it. But, in general, we're adult women; let's stop trivializing ourselves and start being the fabulous, sassy, and sexually empowered women that we are!

That said, I'm all for hotter and more adventurous sex. That's one of the more frequently asked questions I get—how can I make my sex life more adventurous, and how can I spice things up in the bedroom so that things are hot, hot, hot?! As you go through this book, you'll find numerous tips, tricks, and ideas that you can integrate into your sex life, whether you're single and searching, hot and heavy with a monogamous partner, or balancing different lovers as part of your sweltering sex life. Take the parts that seem interesting and fun; leave the ones that are not to your taste; and go forth to have interesting, exciting, and amazing sex as you feel more confident in your sexual prowess.

This book is written for women. All women. Gay, straight, lesbian, queer, bisexual, pansexual, questioning, as well as women who choose not to put labels on themselves. It's for women whose gender has always been in line with the sex they were assigned at birth, and for women who have transitioned into their true gender. It's for girly girls and tomboys, sporty women and butch women. It's for soccer moms, and powerful attorneys, and those who are both. If you identify as a woman in any way, shape, or form, this book is for you. While it has information on partners—on body parts, on how to communicate, and so on, it's for YOU, giving you the information and skills for creating the most confident and sexy-feeling you that you can be.

There's no particular magical trick to being a sexually confident woman, no one way to show that you're an empowered woman. You might be straight, submissive, and empowered. You might be queer, dominant, and empowered. You can be empowered wearing nothing but your birthday suit, a sexy lingerie ensemble, or your favorite sports team's T-shirt. It's crucial that you know that whatever being sexy and feeling empowered looks like to you, that's exactly what you should go for.

I'll step off my soapbox now and let you read. I hope you enjoy the book that's before you, and that you go forth into the world, sexual superheroes, ready to share your sexual confidence with whatever partners may come your way.

1

Romantic Dates

OK. You've picked out an awesome person to date. They're hot and smart, and the chemistry is rocking. Fabulous. Now what?

In this chapter, you'll explore what your ideal date would be like by thinking about:

X--- Your dating style: Are you cool and casual, trendsetting, or classic?

X--- The scene of the crime: Are you in the great outdoors, out on the dance floor, or somewhere a little cozier?

X--- Ending your night: Are you under the stars, with some after-dinner sweets, or taking it on home?

Well, before you can go out to have one of those nights to remember, you should probably ask yourself this question: what's your dating style?

Your Dating Style

Which one sounds like the best fit for the type of date that you'd like to have?

❥ *Cool and Casual*

You want to go somewhere chill and relaxed, where you can get to know each other and there isn't any pressure to perform.

You're laid-back and don't want to have to put on a show for whomever you're dating. In fact, you want to be fun and friendly with them before you hop in the sack, or wherever else the date might be going. Not a problem. These dates are some of the easiest to plan, since you don't want something with too many details or reservations, or with perfect timing that might get messed up. While you probably wouldn't wear a Hawaiian shirt on a date, flip-flops are definitely an option.

When planning a date, you want something that you'll both enjoy, that allows you both to get to know each other more, and that doesn't require any fancy dressing up or plans. Now, you might have been with your partner for years and years, but this type of date is great for striking up more conversation, and who knows: you might discover something completely new and different about them that decades of being together hasn't yet brought up.

Get the Blood Moving

During the thought process, consider activities that are, well, active. Mini-golf, bowling, go-karts, and other such adventures allow for plenty of time to speak to each other, but also give the opportunity for some friendly competition, a little bit of goading back and forth, and interacting with each other in a way that sitting at a high-class bar or watching a movie just wouldn't allow for.

You can always place a bet—whoever wins this game gets to ask a personal question of the other person, or whoever loses has to share their deepest, darkest secret. Of course, bets could always be about who buys the next round, or you could even begin a nice game of strip mini-golf if you're on the course late at night and home is your next step. (Note: I'm not giving you the thumbs-up to be completely naked or have sex on a mini-golf course. That's a whole different type of adventure, and one that you take at your own risk. You can play until someone's about to lose their shirt, then take it home.)

A bonus is that food is often available near all these areas. Granted, the dining options aren't the healthiest (you're not likely to find a kale quinoa salad at the bowling alley), but it's frequently comfort food, which can also spark conversations or at least fill up your belly as you decide what fun and adventurous activity to do next.

Do Some Exploring

Not as sporty? Consider going to the zoo or a local museum to check out an exhibit that you both like. Zoos and museums frequently bring back memories of our childhoods—going on field trips or exploring with our families—so this is a great way to ask questions about what growing up looked like for each of you, yet still be silly as you roar like the lions or pretend to be a T. rex. If you're trying to keep the price down on the date, many museums and zoos have free days (just remember that you may be inundated with children and families who had the exact same idea).

❧ *Trendsetting*

It's see and be seen with you. When you talk about going out for a night on the town, you mean it literally. You want those in the know to know exactly who you are.

If *Cosmo* were a person, you might be her. You're on top of fashion, and maybe a social media guru. You might watch *Entertainment Weekly* like your life depended on it. When someone asks if you know of a good restaurant, you can rattle off a list of all the newest places in town, and you might even know a celebrity chef personally. You understand the point of bottle service and how it works. When you go out on a date, you want to go OUT, with a capital O-U-T.

Points for Planning

These types of dates require a fair amount of planning by one or both interested parties, and aren't ideal if you're looking to fly by the seat of your pants and be spontaneous. This means that you shouldn't wait till the day of the date to start calling around to see if you can get a table. If you're into this kind of date, you probably relish the researching and planning. You might even have reservations at your favorite restaurant as you read this.

But if you're still aspiring to that level of in, or trying to impress a date who relishes hot spots, here are some tips for planning. Check out Facebook and your local newspapers and magazines to find the top restaurants, theaters, and places to be. Yelp can be helpful, too, for deciding whether the new gastro pub is worth the wait and the price … or if it'll be a big, disappointing flop. Ask your friends as well—who just found an awesome new place that they're dying to tell you about, and who knows the word on the street about the bar that just opened with the chef who has a TV show. Once you have a list of places (you can include art galleries, theaters, etc., on this list), it's time to whittle it down.

Keep in mind when your date is. Some places are closed Sundays or Mondays, or are open only for dinner. If you're planning your night on the town for a Friday or Saturday, you may need to try several places to see which ones still have openings, while a Wednesday date at lunch time might afford you more opportunities.

Plan Ahead
Make sure that you check for good deals or packages. Sometimes, a museum or art gallery will pair up with a winery or local restaurant for date-night packages. Not only can you save a few bucks, but you also get to show off your skills of knowing what's going down and how to get in on the action.

If you'd rather pair things up yourself, make sure you know what the parking situation looks like (valet, street parking, meters) and the distance between the locations. You want to ensure that you don't miss your dinner reservation because the art gallery is on the other side of town, and there's no parking anywhere downtown at 7 p.m. on a Saturday night.

A Natural Pairing
Many theaters also have their own restaurant in or near the theater complex, or even as part of the show (dinner theaters are still fabulous, although the food quality may leave a little something

to be desired). When you call to book tickets, ask if they have a restaurant attached or if they can recommend any edgy or trendy places within walking distance.

You Both Should Be on Board

An important part of planning a date of this sort is making sure that both of you are on the same page. You may have reserved bottle services at the hottest club in town, but if you show up in a little black dress and your partner arrives in jeans and a T-shirt, there may be some issues, and not just with getting in the door. Being on top of trends is perfect for some folks, but others may want to relax and get to know you more. Plenty of trendy restaurants have amazing food and a more laid-back atmosphere—patios are especially great for toning things down. If your partner seems a little overwhelmed by dress codes and prices, it might be worth having a conversation about expectations, or find a compromise, like doing the nice restaurant for lunch and something more laid-back for dinner.

♣ *Classic*

Classic, romantic, and even a bit timeless, you want the type of date that will sweep you both off your feet and leave you head over heels at the end of the night.

Calm, classic, and probably a romantic at heart, you don't want to be too casual and leave things to chance, nor do you want to be drinking a martini at the trendiest bar. No siree, you want a date for the ages, one that you can relive over and over, and dissect to see how perfect you two truly are together. We're not quite talking a poodle skirt and saddle shoes, but I bet you wouldn't say no to watching *Casablanca* either.

The Standards Work

You might be the type for whom dinner and a movie are perfect. No, it's not boring; it's a great way to get to know each other by asking questions and feeling each other out (no pun intended), and of course, the movie means that you can hold hands and even cuddle a little during the show. Look for a local drive-in (yes, they still exist in many places) for a truly classic flair. Nothing says old-school romance like making out in the car, fogging up the windows, and then trying to remember what happened in the movie. Or you can go modern and use Netflix or Redbox to watch a movie in the comfort of your home, cozying up on the couch until you both decide how much hanky-panky you want to get into.

Know Your Date's Needs

When you plan a date, make sure that you take your date's dietary needs into account. While the local old-school burger and shake place might sound like a winner, discovering your date is vegan or gluten-free after you get there might shake, rattle, and roll you right out of a romantic evening. Same goes for gauging their movie preferences. If you're going really classic, remember that not everyone is deeply in love with black-and-white films or can read quickly enough to grasp the subtitles on a foreign film.

Do the Twist

There are other fun, more classic options like swing dancing, line dancing, salsa dancing, or square dancing. Most big cities have at least a few options for these kinds of dances, and many of them offer lessons for free or low prices to help you and your date get in the groove before you head out to the floor. Dancing is a fun way to be active in a less intense manner, and it can be incredibly romantic and sexy as you tango or waltz across the floor.

Make-out Point

Already feeling super connected to a lover or loved one? Hop in the car and head to a park, mountaintop, or somewhere else that's mostly deserted for a deliciously devious old-school make-out session in the car. Remember, if the car is a-rockin', don't come a-knockin'! Keep in mind that many parks close at dusk, and you don't want to end up with the police knocking on your steamed-up car windows. While that might be a fun fantasy, getting a real-life ticket for public indecency is not nearly as fun as one might think. Trust me!

The Scene of the Crime

Which of the following sounds most enticing as a location for your date?

> ❥ Getting Close to Nature, *page 14*
>
> ❥ *Showing Off on the Dance Floor or at an Open Mic,* page 16
>
> ❥ Cuddling Up, *page 17*

❥ Getting Close to Nature

You're a nature gal and want to really get wild ... like outdoorsy wild. For some people, the thought of going outdoors on a date creeps them out, but not you. Maybe it's hiking or biking, skiing or snowboarding, or even a sexually charged overnight camping trip—whatever it is, it involves getting in touch with Mother Nature. A lot of people think that reconnecting with the earth helps people to be more grounded and more authentic, and really, is there anything more awesome that you would want on a date than both you and your partner feeling connected together and genuine? Didn't think so.

Take a Lesson from the Scouts and Be Prepared

Because it's nature, it might require a bit more planning than just heading out to dinner. If it's something simple like a hike, then good hiking boots and some water bottles might be all that you need to get going. But if you're planning on hitting some fresh powder or spending the night in the middle of nowhere, you're going to need equipment and supplies. Make sure that you discuss who's responsible for what; it's not fun arriving at your campsite only to discover that neither of you brought food, but together you have enough bug spray to drive mosquitoes extinct. If you don't have the right equipment, the two of you can go together to rent it. You can also check Craigslist to see if you can buy gear on the cheap, or you can borrow it from friends. If you're planning to go on a particular kind of adventure often, purchasing a shiny new snowboard or tent can be a fun date in itself.

When Mother Nature Has Other Plans

Keep in mind that sometimes nature won't behave the way you want it to, so have a backup plan. It could mess with your date mojo if you get stuck on a snowy road or if there's a hailstorm in the middle of your hike. Make sure you check the weather and have a plan B that you can readily execute. Keep in mind that things like poison ivy and an allergic reaction to a bug bite might throw a wrench in your naturist lovemaking plans; be ready to be supportive of each other and go with the flow. Even if things don't go as planned, being laid-back will let you enjoy your nature-filled experience and bond over that beautiful sunset or the Black Diamond slope that you both just crushed—or didn't.

❥ *Showing Off on the Dance Floor or at an Open Mic*

You've got some moves and want to be seen. It's time for you to get out there and strut your stuff. I'm not saying that you need to be the main event everywhere you go, but you're chock-full of energy, and want to be out and about with people.

Getting Close in the Club

Maybe hitting the club is where it's at. If you like some eyes to be on you, the dance floor is a great place to get that. You and your partner can get close as your bodies are rubbing on the dance floor, and you want to show off your slick moves as you salsa the night away.

So This Couple Walks into a Bar

The club might not be your thing, and dancing might not be your style. Perhaps going to a comedy club on a date would allow you to be out and about, let your hair down, and have some great laughs. Maybe going to an improv group, where you can shout things out, would help you to feel engaged. You could even show off your own chops at an open mic night or a karaoke bar. If that's a bit too much, there's a comeback trend of murder-mystery theater that involves the audience in solving the crime, letting you be part of the show while still getting to relax and kick back.

It Takes Two to Tango

The trick here is to make sure that your date feels the same way. You might be an extrovert of the highest degree (or even an introvert with extrovert tendencies), but your date might be a homebody who would rather just blend into the background. Forcing someone who wants to be more chill and quiet into the limelight can be a super-stressful experience for them. If your date's not quite thrilled with the prospect of showing off their moves on the dance floor or is terrified of being called on at a show, give a little compassion and come up with a compromise that fulfills your love of going out on the town with their need for something more laid-back and relaxed.

❥ *Cuddling Up*

You COULD go out and about. You COULD see and be seen. You COULD escape to the mountains or the beach. But why would you when you could be somewhere that lets you get cozy with your date? Of course, this could be as simple as going to you or your date's place to veg out on the couch or snuggle in bed. Never fear. There are lots of other options to make things a little more interesting.

Climate-Controlled Stargazing

Check out the planetarium at the local museum. Beautiful stars, comfy seats, and the chance to get close with your date. Obviously, a regular movie might work just as well: look for a theater that has seats with movable arms. Just raise the arm, scoot over, and you get a first-rate movie experience with popcorn, surround sound, and as much cuddling as you want.

Plush Picnic

Have a picnic in the park or even just in your backyard. Bring a comfy blanket and maybe some pillows for your head (or other body parts that might need some softness). Set yourself up where you can see the sunset if you're rocking out on an evening, or just lie in the sun or in the shade—wherever you want—if you're on a fun and relaxing afternoon date. A cuddly nap in the park is hard to beat.

Someone Else's Couch

You can also find a coffee shop or bar with comfy couches and stuffed chairs that hosts an open mic night or local musicians. Often free, or at least cheap, these places offer a space where you can cuddle up with a drink or cup of joe while enjoying poetry, music, and more. Just don't get too frisky; save that hands-on attention for back at your place!

Ending Your Night

It's the end of the night (or end of the afternoon or even morning, depending on when you decided to have your fabulous date). It's time to think about closing the deal.

Which of these seems the most like what you'd want to do at the end of a date?

- ❥ *Starstruck Views, page 18*
- ❥ *Delicious Dessert and Drinks, page 20*
- ❥ *Heading on Home for Cuddling, page 21*

❥ *Starstruck Views*

For many people, the classic idea of a couple stretched out on the hood of their car or on a blanket on the top of a hill is as good as it gets. Commercials have co-opted this concept to sell everything from jewelry to cars, and why? Because there's just something so touching about enjoying the beautiful sky with someone whose company you relish.

Chart the Stars

If you like that type of sweet and slightly sensual end to the evening, maybe do some research on the best places to see the stars — if you live in an urban area, you'll probably have to go outside the city limits to get the best views. With most cars, you can just lie on the hood, but if you have a pickup truck or SUV with a back gate, then toss in some pillows and maybe a light blanket in case it gets cold. If the car isn't ideal for lying on, you definitely want to grab a few blankets and pillows for lying on the grass or beach. One blanket can go underneath you and one can go on top in case it gets chilly (or you want to get a little frisky and don't want to risk public exposure).

Make sure you keep in mind any local laws (like a park's closing time) and where you are (you don't want to get in trouble for trespassing when you're trying to end a romantic date). As long as you're in little to no risk of getting a ticket, making out under the stars can be super sweet.

Think Ahead

If you think there might be even a small chance of some sexual action happening, make sure you're prepared with anything you might need, like safe-sex supplies and lube. You don't want a romantic moment to turn into either "I want to get it on, but we can't" or "we just got it on without adequate protection, and now I'm going to spend the next several weeks worried about STIs, pregnancy, or both." Be prepared for the best, and even if you don't make it to that stage, you'll be covered. Literally. Also, consider bringing bug spray. Mosquito bites on your naughty bits are no fun at all. Promise.

❧ *Delicious Dessert and Drinks*

Maybe you're not quite sure yet if you want to go for a sexual situation with your date, or maybe you have a craving for chocolate that just won't leave you alone. Either way, it's totally kosher to finish your date night on a sweet note with some drinks, dessert, or even both.

Keep with the Theme

Depending on what your date was like, you could go to a dessert-specific restaurant, stop by a mom-and-pop shop for a slice of pie, drop by a dive bar for a pint, or imbibe a glass of your favorite vintage at a local wine bar. Wherever you decide to end your evening, this allows you to wind things down and check in with each other about how you're feeling. You can laugh about amusing things that happened, plan your next date, or, if it comes down to it, discuss whether you even feel any chemistry. Perhaps you might even head to option C from here, if that's what you so decide.

Desserts Don't Have to Be the Only Sweet Thing

Just because you decide to end your date this way doesn't mean that sex is off the table. You could head home and start doing the mattress mambo now, or you could let the tension build for another date or two (or more) before you decide to move on to anything. Check in with yourself and what *you* want. Are you feeling frisky, fried, or meh?

If you do decide to end the date there and then, you need to decide how you feel about an end-of-the-evening kiss. Sure, you can wait until the last minute, but having an idea of how you feel about locking lips before you actually do will give you a way to gauge what to do in the actual moment. If you aren't feeling it, it's kinder to avoid a misleading kiss than give in to one because you feel that it's the right thing to do at the end of a date. The thing to do is whatever you want to have happen, conventions be damned!

❥ *Heading on Home for Cuddling*

OK. You're ready to head home and see what (or even *who*) might come from your date's festivities. You have a choice: your place or theirs (unless you already live together, and in that case, your decision has already been made for you). Once you get there, then you need to think about what you're interested in doing.

Nothing Is a Sure Thing

Just because you're heading home, where there's likely a bed, doesn't mean that anything of a sexual nature has to happen. You get to decide exactly what you feel good about doing. That could be anything from making out to cuddling on the couch, any type of sexual interaction from manual stimulation to oral sex to penetration. It's all on the table, but it's important to communicate your wants to your date. If your date is ready for making out and you're ready for a few hours of sex, that's where miscommunications can occur. The bus/train/car ride home is a great time to get some sexually charged conversation going—sharing what you'd like them to do to you, or what you'd like to do to them, lays it all out so you both know where you're going to stand … or sit … or lie … or, well, whatever works for you. It may feel a little awkward to get the conversation going, but being upfront and honest can save you from an even more awkward conversation later.

Chapter

Fantastic Foreplay

Ah, foreplay. That good ole pretty dang important part of sex play that frequently doesn't get as much lip service as it deserves. People frequently ask, "How much foreplay needs to happen?" as if they're going to set an egg timer exactly to the minute, or even second, and as soon as it dings, move on to the main event. Au contraire, my friends. Foreplay has no magical number that determines how long it should last. It's different for each individual, and while in general, the rule is that if you think you've done enough foreplay, do some more, a portion of the population doesn't need much in the way of foreplay. Again, communication is crucial in figuring it out.

In this chapter you'll find out:

> **X**--- How much foreplay works for you: Super quick, middle of the road, or lots and lots.

X--- What gets your motor going: Making out, handiwork, or oral.

X--- How to connect with your inner sex goddess by deciding whether you like lingerie, lighting, or just your bare body best!

How Much Foreplay Do You Really Want?

When it comes to the amount of time that you want to spend on foreplay, which of the following best describes you?

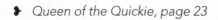

➤ *Queen of the Quickie, page 23*

➤ *More Middle of the Road, page 24*

➤ *Proud Pillow Princess, page 26*

➤ *Queen of the Quickie*

You're one of those women who can go from zero to sixty in the blink of an eye. Perhaps this is because you naturally have such a high sex drive that you're raring to go, or maybe you spend your days giving yourself fabulous foreplay with dirty thoughts about things to come (literally). Whatever it is, you're sick of being told that all women need hours and hours of foreplay when what you really want is more of a wham, bam, thank you ma'am.

Good for You!

First of all, that's absolutely OK and normal. Unfortunately, when people try to give sex advice with the idea that ALL women like or dislike something, or that ALL women need or don't need something, those who don't fit the blanket statement get left high and dry. If you're perfectly fine with quickies that don't require much foreplay at all, or you prefer to just dive into the main event, then good for you for knowing your own mind and body.

Make Sure It's Good for Everybody

However, it is important to note that although YOU may not need or want more foreplay, your partner might. Regardless of gender, your partner may really enjoy different types of foreplay, and they might be a bit put off by you saying that it's not on the menu that night (of course, they might also just say "awesome" and begin with the main course, which would be great for you both). Make sure that you communicate to them that it's YOU who doesn't necessarily need or want that extra warm-up time, but that has nothing to do with how you feel about them. Many people equate foreplay with caring for each other, so you may want to offer up more foreplay for them if THEY feel that they need or want it.

Finding a happy compromise is the name of the game here. You could always alternate between fast-and-fun quickies and longer sex sessions, or you could provide the foreplay that they desire before moving on to what you're really wanting. Just make sure to keep up with the communication, and you should be good to go!

✦ *More Middle of the Road*

You like having a good amount of foreplay before you get down to business, but too much foreplay and you start to get a little antsy. You fall right in the middle, so for you, figuring out the happy medium of foreplay is what it'll take to keep you sexually satisfied.

Taking It Down a Notch

If you're getting TOO much foreplay from your partner (yes, this can happen, especially when a partner who's eager to please reads an article that says hours of foreplay make every woman sexually happy), the task at hand is communicating to them that you appreciate how much foreplay they're providing while letting them know that you're so incredibly turned on by the first ten to twenty minutes of foreplay that you just don't need the rest and are aching to get to the main event. Remember to throw some compliments in there, especially about the parts and amounts of the foreplay that you're enjoying. You don't want to hurt their feelings or somehow accidentally convince them that you don't need any foreplay at all.

Turning It Up a Notch

On the other hand, what if you have a partner who just isn't giving you enough foreplay? You should think a bit about what kind of foreplay you'd like to add that you're not getting, and while you don't need to have an exact number (thirteen minutes of fingering, please!), a time frame might give them some ideas of what your needs are. For example, you might say that you're happy with the amount of hot kissing and making out that the two of you currently do, but that the two minutes of receiving oral sex is not quite getting you to where you need to be. Saying that ten minutes of their amazing mouth would really turn you on so that you're ready for what's next is a lot clearer than just saying, "I need more foreplay."

Finding Their Fit

Don't forget that our partners have their own foreplay wants and needs. Make sure that the conversation you have about your own needs and desires for foreplay also gives them time to share their wants and needs. If the two of you are already on the same page, that's wonderful, and you can go forth into sexy time. If you're at different places of need for amounts of foreplay (both giving and receiving), come up with some compromises that will allow you both to feel that you're getting your needs met.

❥ *Proud Pillow Princess*

When people talk about the need for hours and hours of foreplay (albeit a bit hyperbolically), they're speaking your language. Sure, the idea of getting it on without much action first might interest you, but you know your body like the back of your hand, inside and out. You crave, want, and NEED a significant amount of foreplay before any other sexual activity takes place. In fact, sometimes you might even be happier with only "foreplay" happening, as it can be just as exciting as, if not even more satisfying than, the main event.

Getting Yours

That's great that you know your own needs. The challenging part is ensuring that those needs get met. Sadly, many mainstream depictions of sexual interactions portray women who need only to be looked at with a smoldering gaze before their panties are in a pile on the floor and they are ready to be taken. You have the (potentially difficult) task in front of you of disillusioning your current partner (or even potential partners) of this myth and training them on how to best get you ready for whatever the main event might be.

Know What to Ask For

Think about what foreplay means to you: Is it kissing? Oral sex? Fingering action? Cuddling together on the couch? Reading erotica out loud to each other? Once you have a more solid understanding of what foreplay means to you, you'll be better able to share what foreplay needs to look like with your partner. Specifics are good—instead of saying, "I'd like to be kissed for a longer period of time," you might consider saying something like, "When you make out with me for like ten minutes, I start to get REALLY turned on."

Again, communication is important, not only in letting your partner know about your needs, but doing it in a way that assures them that you're attracted to them and that they're not doing anything wrong. You want them to feel excited and engaged about doing more foreplay, not like they're bad at sex. You can also give updates throughout the foreplay about how much more you're getting turned on, how aroused you are, and so on, to let them know that the extra work they're doing is paying off. Additionally, make sure that extra foreplay is a two-way street if they enjoy it as well; don't make them do all the work if they too might enjoy a little extra oral or handiwork as part of your sexual play.

Coming to a Compromise
You might also want to discuss with your partner ways that you might compromise—you might not always have the time for them to go down on you for forty-five minutes before you move on to intercourse. Consider planning a foreplay-heavy sexual interaction once a week, while having more of a quickie (maybe just ten to fifteen minutes of oral sex, or just a few minutes of making out) once a week, so that you both can get what you most crave without always having to put aside two hours for sex.

What Gets Your Motor Going?

Foreplay is kind of a misnomer, implying that certain things are just precursors and are not actually sex. I mean, really, any sexual activity can be done as foreplay, as the main event, as an afterthought, or even as the only thing happening that night. That being said, in truth we tend to think of a few specific things as foreplay, and if you know exactly what it is that revs you up, you can let your partner know, leading to an even more fantastic time in the bedroom.

As you think about it, what really turns you on and gets you ready for going even hotter and heavier? Maybe you are:

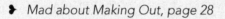

- ❥ *Mad about Making Out, page 28*
- ❥ *Hooked on Handiwork, page 29*
- ❥ *Orally Predisposed, page 31*

❥ Mad about Making Out

Ah, the somewhat lost art of the good make-out session. For some reason, although it was all the rage in high school when it was a huge part of our intimate times with our partners, it has somehow lost much of its magic and allure. Many people are lucky if they can get in a few hot kisses before their clothes are on the floor and lips have moved on to other areas.

Slow and Steady

Many sex therapists, especially when working with clients who feel that sex has gotten stale or routine, encourage them to give up other sexual activities for a while and just go back to making out, exploring each other's faces, lips, necks, ears, collar bones, and so on, with their lips, and letting their hands wander all over each other … but just above the waist. While many people think this sounds silly, it's an incredibly effective way to reengage with someone. Making out allows you to connect in a whole different way than you might while doing the mattress mambo. You can rediscover some of your lover's erogenous zones that you might have forgotten about (or never even found in the first place), and they get to do the same for you and your body.

There's also something a bit hot about the idea of being all kinds of hot and bothered but having to stay above the belt. Maybe it takes us back to high school when we weren't yet ready for other activities, or maybe it's just the urge to want what we can't have that makes it that much hotter. Either way, you may find that if you and your partner just focus on kissing and making out for a while, it'll free up other areas of your sex drive and leave you both all wound up and ready to go.

The Right Time
If you love making out and your partner is ambivalent about it but will do it to make you happy, you could consider setting a time frame; making out through the next four songs on the iPod or until the oven dings. That way, the person who isn't all about making out doesn't feel that they have to perform for hours on end, and you know that you're definitely getting at least the minimum fulfillment of your make-out needs and wants.

❧ Hooked on Handiwork
Fingering, finger banging, handiwork—whatever name you have for it, you love it when your partner gets all kinds of handsy with you. From gently stroking your labia and clitoris with lubed-up

fingers (lube can make all the difference) to slooooowly sliding inside you until you can barely breathe from anticipation, having some manual action between your legs is the type of foreplay that makes you ready to jump your partner's bones.

Opening Act or Main Event?

For some people, manual stimulation is definitely foreplay and is always a precursor, never the main event. Others enjoy it as the highlight of their interaction, whether or not there are other activities coming down the pipeline. For many people, manual stimulation is a much more enjoyable sensation than penetration with a penis or dildo, and can certainly be more sexually fulfilling, resulting in orgasms more frequently. Manual stimulation can involve just fingers, or also a vibrator for the clit that could be exclusively external stimulation or might include penetration of the vagina (or anus) as well.

Talk to the Hand

Even with handiwork, it's important to communicate with your partner about what that looks like to you, and how you want it to happen. A lot of partners are super excited about hot fingering action, but you might want them to stroke around your vulva until you're absolutely begging them to put their finger(s) inside you. On the other hand, you might be ready to go with your favorite vibrator to take care of external stimulation, and just want them to slip and slide right in. If they're penetrating you, make sure that they know if you just want them inside you being perfectly still, if you want their fingers straight or curved, if you want them going in and out—the better you can communicate your needs and wants to your partner, the more likely it is that they'll be fulfilled.

Sometimes Dull Is Good

If they're using their fingers on or around your vulva, or inside your vagina or anus, make sure there are no sharp edges, rough hang nails, and so on. That tissue is easily snagged and cut during this type of sexual activity. People often cut their nails before sex to get rid of ragged edges, but it doesn't occur to them that unless they ALSO file their nails, they're now putting freshly cut, super-sharp nails into their partner's most delicate areas. If their nails are indeed too sharp or ragged, or have a hangnail, consider asking your partner to use a latex, nitrile, or vinyl glove. It'll keep things nice and slippery as well as protect your skin down there from any uncomfortable and accidental cuts.

❧ *Orally Predisposed*

Mmm. The feeling of your partner's mouth pressed up against your vulva, their tongue working its magic as your back arches up from the bed, just can't be beat. While of course some women flat out don't enjoy receiving oral sex (and of course, that's absolutely normal and A-OK), there are in fact many who adore the feeling of their lover eating them out. Cunnilingus (oral sex on a vulva) is a sexual activity that many women can climax from, making it a great foreplay (or after-play!) option, especially if they're not able to orgasm from other types of sexual activities like intercourse and/or penetration.

Relax about Receiving

Some women who enjoy receiving cunnilingus are also concerned about being on the receiving end. Some think that it seems selfish, but it's not any more selfish than when your partner receives oral sex—it's 100 percent acceptable for you to lie back and let yourself go as you enjoy yourself sexually. There's NOTHING wrong with that.

Others may be concerned about the taste. But if you're in good health (i.e., no infections or other medical issues), you taste the way you're supposed to. If you're truly concerned, stay away from cream (and most dairy), garlic, broccoli, and asparagus, and make friends with your favorite citrusy fruits and juices like pineapple, oranges, limes, and lemons if you want to taste slightly sweeter.

Another concern some have is that your partner thinks cunnilingus is gross. I have to tell you, one of the most frequently asked questions that I get is, "How come my girlfriend/wife/partner won't let me go down on her? I think it's so incredibly sexy to eat her out, but she keeps pushing me away." While yes, some people may not enjoy giving cunnilingus, the vast majority do. If your partner says that they don't like it, you can always ask why and try to troubleshoot, but think first if they actually said they didn't like it or if you're putting words in their mouth.

Shower Before Showtime

If you're concerned with your smell or taste (or their smell or taste), or cleanliness in general before oral sex, add hopping in the shower together to rub each other up and soap each other down as part of your foreplay routine. Since you both just showered together, you both know that you're fresh and clean, and that can sometimes help your mind relax more to lie back and enjoy receiving cunnilingus. Stay away from frou-frou soaps with fragrance; use pH-balanced soaps or ones that are slightly basic (less acidic) if you're soaping up below the belt!

Take Your Time

You may need to let your partner know if you need more or less time in the oral sex department. Mainstream media and mainstream porn tend to show cunnilingus that lasts all of a minute or two, but many women want more than that. It's absolutely OK to let your partner know that you love what they're doing to you, that it really turns you on, and that you need about another fifteen or twenty minutes of them doing what they're doing for you to either climax or to be ready to go on to the next activity.

If you know you need a little bit longer for cunnilingus, consider getting into a position that's comfortable for you both for the majority of the time, and then as you get close, you can switch into the position in which you like to end. This way, your partner's head and neck don't get too tired out and you're still getting your requisite amount of oral sex.

Further Reading and Experimentation

If you want to learn more about oral sex, female anatomy, and positions for cunnilingus, check out my book *Oral Sex That'll Blow Her Mind: An Illustrated Guide to Giving Her Amazing Orgasms*. The whole book focuses solely on cunnilingus and what you can do to make it the best possible. You can also feel free to experiment, and you should make sure to check back in with your partner to give them feedback on what you liked and want them to do again, as well as telling them what wasn't quite as exciting. As with all types of sexual activity, make sure that you're on top of your communication, giving positive feedback, and coming to a middle ground around things that you don't just magically agree on.

Connecting with Your Inner Sex Goddess!

People are always talking about sex tips—how to be the sexiest, how to be the best at sex, and so on. However, for the most part, there's no one magical tip that works for everyone. Different strokes for different folks (pun intended), and all of that. That's fine and dandy, but there's one tip that works for everyone, regardless of their age, experience, gender, orientation, relationship status, and so on. That tip? Confidence and enthusiasm are sexy. Period. If you feel good about you—about how you look, how you feel, and how excited you are for whatever sexual adventure is about to happen, then you're far more likely to be viewed as sexy by others.

Granted, that seems like a simple piece of advice that's so boiled down that it means nothing. That may be true, but connecting with your inner sex goddess (I promise, everyone has one) is going to make you better in bed, for yourself and for your partner. It will.

So how does one do that? It's incredibly complicated. Women are socialized in our society to feel that they need to conform to a certain look, a certain style, even a certain way of being sexy. Even most of the "stereotypically beautiful" women, including supermodels, spend a good deal of their time picking apart what's wrong with them rather than celebrating all the amazing and beautiful parts of their body. If you go into sex trying to hide your body, or with the idea that you aren't worth it, then the sex is not going to be great—all those feelings are going to be weighing you down the whole time, and rather than concentrating on pleasure (giving, receiving, or both), you'll be spending your time wondering if your partner has noticed your mole/your fat/your skinniness/your tan line/your hair, or mulling over whether this is pity sex, or if it'll ever happen again, or why such a sexy person wants to sleep with you. With all those things running through your head, is it any wonder that it's hard to focus on being in the moment? So let's break it down based on three things that can help you feel sexy and powerful.

When you think about looking and being your best in the boudoir, which of the following resonates the most?

❥ *Stunning Your Lover with Your Looks, page 35*

❥ *Being Cast in the Perfect Lighting, page 38*

❥ *Walking in Like You Own the Place, page 40*

❥ *Stunning Your Lover with Your Looks*

Lingerie is an industry. Long before there were silky bras, beautiful bustiers, and perfect panties, people were still having ridiculously awesome sex. So what is it about our society that makes people feel that they have to spend a fortune on garments that contain the smallest bits of cloth? No easy answer to that one, but many women feel that they can't be sexy unless they look like a Victoria Secret's model, and that just isn't true.

Confidence with Lingerie

To start with, wear what makes you feel sexy. Again, that's what makes YOU feel sexy, not what your partner will find sexy, or what the TV tells you is sexy. Do you feel like a lioness ready to take down her prey when you're wearing that old college T-shirt and yoga pants? Then don't abandon them for a negligee that makes you feel timid and overexposed—wear the yoga pants. Really. Do you feel sexiest when you wear nothing under your clothes, and go from fully clothed to nothing but nude? If so, stick with the commando, and go that way. Your partner's going to think you're sexy if YOU think and feel that you're sexy, lingerie or otherwise.

Lingerie as Lingerie

This is all fine and dandy if you don't feel sexy in lingerie, but what if you do? That's great too — it's all about finding the right look, feel, and fit for you that stays within your budget. Who knows, maybe you have hundreds or thousands to blow on beautiful and flimsy garments. If so, then off you go. However, if like most folks, you can afford a few pieces that make you feel beautiful, then the key is finding those pieces.

Down Below

Thongs: people love them or hate them. If you fall into the former camp, then there are so many adorable thongs and G-strings (there's no real difference between the two, other than a few centimeters of fabric) to choose from, and they can range from about $5 at places like Target to hundreds of dollars at high-end stores, and everything in between. You can get cotton thongs, silk thongs, lace thongs — you name it. Some people love the look of thongs, or they like the stimulation of their bits, or both. Other people find them a bit comfortable — if you fall into that group, read on!

For those of us not in the thong camp, another super-sexy item is the newly popular boy short. Why so popular? Because boy shorts are still sexy and don't remind folks of the white cotton panties preferred by schoolgirls and grandmothers (although if that's your thing, then power to you as well!), yet still have the comfort that some don't seem to find in thongs. Plus, everyone's butt looks good in boy shorts, whether you have very little in your trunk or were the inspiration for "Baby Got Back." Like thongs, they come in various materials, patterns, and colors.

Up Top

So we've got the bottom half covered—what about what goes on top? For some, a sexy bra is the easy answer. Again, these can come in a huge variety of styles from full coverage to demi-cup, strapless and backless, even sports bras (which can be very sexy to some folks). Find a bra that's comfortable, unless you're going to make it your "sex-time-only bra," in which case comfort doesn't have to be an issue. Make sure you try them on—the sizes fit differently for different brands, and even in the same brand from style to style. If you've never been fit for a bra, I highly encourage you to go to your local higher-end bra shop and have someone do it for you. It's free and usually more accurate than any store I've been to in a mall or open-air shopping center. Knowing your correct sizes can significantly change your confidence and sexy-feeling during bra wearing.

Getting Tucked In

Want a little more coverage? A little more boost? A little more to take off? You could go the way of a bustier (what you find in lingerie stores) or a corset (real corsets have hefty boning, are more expensive, and are sometimes harder to find). This may tuck you in a little in the middle and also add some oomph to your breasts. If you want the girls free to hang out in a sexy bra but want that support for your middle, they make half-bustiers/corsets called cinchers that go below your breasts. Teddies were popular in the 1980s, but seem to have gone out of style, although you can still find them some places—they look like loose leotards made of more whimsical material.

Nighty Nightie

If you want to go classic, negligees are like lingerie nightgowns and can be full coverage or see-through, and go to the floor or just below your butt cheeks (these ones are usually called baby dolls), and many of them, especially in a larger size, have built-in support or even underwire cups, while some are more flimsy and just for show. Some come with matching panties and/or robes, and others are stand-alone.

❥ *Being Cast in the Perfect Lighting*

So many people, especially women, dread being naked in front of a lover, a partner, even a one-night stand. People joke that the first step of sex is to turn the lights out; many women have never had a sexual experience with any lights on, much less in full light. The trick to getting out of the dark? Finding the light that works best for you.

While sex in the dark CAN be fun as one of many options, limiting yourself to always being in the shadows is just that—limiting. The view of bodies during sex is another enticing turn-on for all those involved, and being confident enough to show off your body in the most flattering light projects that assuredness, which can be incredibly arousing, both for the confident individual and for the one watching that confidence shine.

Ditch the Standard

Most indoor lights are fluorescent, which is probably the least flattering type of light available, ever. Fluorescent light bleaches color from construction paper on billboards because it's so harsh, and emphasizes little things like blemishes, while also doing weird things like changing skin tones. Although this type of lighting is fine for making your bed and choosing tomorrow's outfit, it's not ideal for gently lighting your skin while you're getting ready to get it on.

NOT the Brightest Bulb in the Box

Consider some other options. One of the easiest is to replace the existing bulbs in your current light fixtures with soft white, non-fluorescent bulbs, or even fun-colored bulbs. Red can have a passionate fiery feel, while blue can be more calming. You can also eschew the built-in light fixture and rely on small or large lamps. Then you can change lampshades to light the room the way you'd like. Just please don't throw fabric over a light to soften the lighting—that's a major fire hazard, and nothing is more of a sexual buzzkill than the sound of sirens and alarms going off.

Lighting a Flame, Literally

More into natural lighting? Candles are tried and true, and everyone looks fabulous in candlelight. Massage candles are soy based and can be used for lighting to start, and then as melted wax massage oil during the fun. You can use tiny tea lights, or large glass jar candles, and everything in between. Choose a scent that's sensual to you and not too overpowering; you don't want to be thinking about warm baked cookies while you're doing the deed. Something to keep in mind; keep candles away from pets and flammable objects.

Be a Sun Goddess

A final option, depending on when you're planning the mattress mambo, is the use of good ole natural daylight. Granted, if your window faces a busy street, you might want to invest in some nice shades or sheer fabric to put over the window. However, soft daylight, especially on an overcast day, is some of the most flattering light out there, all for the ridiculously amazing price of FREE.

So yes, you can have fabulously flattering light in the bedroom that encourages you to flaunt your curves. And maybe one day—once you've gained the confidence that comes with loving who you are and how you look, however that may be—perhaps you won't even need to prelight your bedroom. You'll be able to go into any situation with any lighting and rock out like the wonderful sex goddess that you know that you are!

❥ *Walking in Like You Own the Place*

Stop for a moment and think about what you're really good at, the thing that makes you most confident. Perhaps it's your superior negotiating skills, or your fabulous gardening green thumb, or your amazing ability to interact with people. Now, think about how wonderful it would be if you could replicate that confidence when you saunter into the bedroom, raring to go.

Conning Confidence

The number one trick to this type of sexual confidence is the idea of faking it until you make it. Does this sound a bit silly? Yes … but let's be honest, sex is a little silly. We all have bodies that are a little funny, and we make odd noises, and we have odd names for our body parts. No one is naturally born with the sexual prowess of a sex god or goddess; we all put on a front around sexuality, a facade that implies that we know what we're doing. Only once we put on that front and gain practice, experience, and maybe even a bit of sexual humility (we've all had the ridiculously awkward sexual experiences that end with a good laugh and hilarious story to be told later among friends) do we become sexually confident and full of those bedroom skills that we perhaps only pretended to have before.

Now, I'm not saying to go into the bedroom being a cocky asshole (pun intended) know-it-all. That won't serve anyone. You still have to be ready to communicate your wants and needs, and to listen to the wants and needs of your partner. That being said, there's a huge difference between saying, "I'm so excited to learn what gets you going and show you what works for me," and, "I have no idea what I'm doing, but guess I'll just do it."

Role-Play Your Role Models a Little Bit

Think about your favorite badass role model. Beyoncé, Marlene Dietrich, Gloria Steinem, bell hooks, Mae West, Pink; you name her, and she can be a powerful woman who's your role model. Now reflect on what makes her so amazing and powerful—is it her calmness, powerful presence, sultry voice, witty comebacks? Take a moment to figure out how to integrate that trait into your bedroom banter. Walk in, strike a pose, and say, "Hey there, sailor," or do a little dance that you know will draw your partner's eyes to your favorite body parts. Maybe it's more cerebral, like talking about social or gender theory while you unbutton your lover's shirt. Or it may even just be walking in and telling them what you want them to do, and that you want it now.

The goal is for you to figure out your own shtick—what it is that boosts your sexual confidence and makes you ready to walk in and take the reins. Getting there is usually a process, and borrowing a few tricks from our favorite folks never hurt us. Just don't get too much into character (unless you're doing a role-play that involves that), because you might end up confusing your lover more than showing them your confident side.

Chapter

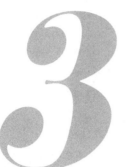

Naked Time: Exploring Bodies

It's that time. You're starting to think about a certain person in a certain way, and you're on your way to getting naked and touching each other in some deliciously delightful places. In this chapter, you can:

X--- Find adventure in the erogenous zones such as lovely lips, delicious nipples, and below the belt.

X--- Survey sensual areas like the neck, the thighs, or anywhere else that's often overlooked.

Adventures in the Erogenous Zones!

What do you think when you hear the term *erogenous zones*? Most people immediately think penis or vulva, but tend to forget about all the other deliciousness going on. You have numerous nerve endings connected to pretty much every single part of your body. We'll get into some of the even less commonly thought of areas in the next section, but let's talk sensual zones. Where do you want to go first?

- ❥ *Luscious Lips, page 43*
- ❥ *Delicious Nipples, page 44*
- ❥ *Below the Belt, page 45*

❥ *Luscious Lips*

Your lips (the ones above your waist … yes, the ones on your face, not between your legs) are full of nerves just aching to be stimulated. Kissing is great, but rather than just a few pecks here and there or some tonsil hockey happenings, consider making love to your lover's lips. Gently caress and stroke them with your own lips, with a finger, with a dripping ice cube—feel free to get super creative. Nibble them nicely … or naughtily, however you (and they) prefer. Catch their bottom lip between your teeth and pull back gently until you hear your partner moan. Don't just kiss 'em and leave 'em alone—show their lips, and yours, that you know exactly how delightful they can feel when they're properly used.

❥ *Delicious Nipples*

And how about the nipples? True, not everyone loves to have their nipples touched, but a lot more people do than you might think. While we tend to think of women's nipples as sensual, they're usually just a quick stop for a little "come in Tokyo, come in Moscow" radio-dial action on the way down the treasure trail, and when it comes to men's nipples? Pshaw! You'd think that they didn't exist for all the lack of lip service we give them.

Don't Just Do a Flyby

No matter your sex or gender, nipples are chock-full of nerve endings (unless you've had surgery that might affect this), and many of these endings wind up ending right between your legs. So playing with the nipples and giving them a little bit of air time, rather than just dusting over them on the way to the genitals, is going to get both of you much more fired up.

Start Slow

Don't just go in for "the kill" (a.k.a. the radio-dial twist—which, to be honest, few people like just by itself). Endear yourself to those passionate peaks. Circle around them, explore them. Use your fingers, your tongue, some feathery goodness, ice cubes, whipped cream—anything you can think of, give it a go, and really get to know both sets of nipples, yours AND theirs. You can play with your own nipples to give your partner a little bit of a sensual show, and then return the focus back to theirs. Flick nicely, pinch a little, lick, suck, nuzzle, blow on, circle, stroke—figure out what feels best, and do a lot of that sandwiched between a bit more exploring. Once they're even more revved and raring to go, then, and only then, should you desert these mountainous peaks and travel farther south.

❧ *Below the Belt*

Now you're finally nearing what you might have thought of as your goal all along. Do NOT get too excited yet. We're not going to dive in for the cherry on top too soon—there are so many fun and delicious things to do between the legs before you start focusing solely on the vulva or on the penis and testicles.

Spend some time on the pubic bone. Everyone has some epic sensations running just below this area—some folks may call it a "mons pubis," and others have different names for it, but all that you need to know is that it's awesome, and highly sensitive. Run your palms on it, lightly at first, and then put a bit more pressure on it, pulling up toward the stomach. Now, don't press too hard, but what you're doing is stimulating the nerve endings for the genitals in a new and unique way. Pretty cool, right? In fact, much of our sexual sensation occurs INSIDE the body, instead of just on the outside! Now use your fingers and gently trail them along the areas where the legs meet the rest of the body, along the outside of the outer lips or at the base of the penis where it connects to the body. These areas are highly sensitive, and because they're frequently ignored during sexual playtime, they're highly primed with some stimulation. Give it to them before you continue on.

Survey Sensual Areas Often Overlooked!

You little tease, you love giving your partner all kinds of pleasure, especially anything not traditionally connected to the genital region. Good for you—it takes some terrific talent to hold back from the main course in order to tenderize and tantalize your willing victim.

Now, you've probably heard this fact before, but maybe not in such a sensual and sexual context. The skin is your largest organ. This means that anywhere you touch is going to end up with tons of nerve endings firing back pleasure signals to the brain saying "Holy cow, this feels amazing!" Yeah, sure, the genitals may have more nerve endings per square inch, but since when did we decide to take quantity over quality? Touch can feel absolutely amazing wherever it is, and it's up to you to figure out the spots that drive your partner absolutely wild and vice versa! Where would you love your partner to spend some extra time tonight?

❥ *The Neck, page 46*

❥ *The Thighs, page 47*

❥ *Everywhere Else, page 47*

❥ *The Neck*

The neck is the easy one. Ears too. Almost everyone (the key word here is almost; it's OK if you or your partner is not part of the majority here) enjoys having their neck or ears touched, nibbled, licked, and so on, so go for it. Notice that I said nibbled and not eaten like a rabid dog. People sometimes get a little too aggressive here, and that can result in unintended hickies. Given that turtlenecks are out of style, this could cause some awkward moments. Rather than suck away like a … well … sucker fish, or bite like your life depended on it, gently lick the neck and blow on the area for a little temperature play. Nibble with your lips gently to give them a tingle or two down the spine. Softly bite their earlobes—this area is much harder (though not impossible) to accidentally bruise. Use your fingers, your tongue, your lips, the tip of your nose—think outside the box and nuzzle up to them in various ways.

❧ *The Thighs*

Once you've taken care of the neck or ears, it's time to explore other oft-neglected areas that can be a huge turn-on. Many people love having the area on and around their hip bones kissed, and this is a great way to tease your partner, since it feels so close to their genital area without getting into the "it" zone. The same goes for licking, kissing, nibbling, and sucking the inside of the thighs. There are tons of nerve endings, so close to the hot zone, but it's definitely a bit of a tease because you're not diving in to the action quite yet.

❧ *Everywhere Else*

Think about places that don't receive touch regularly—try kissing from the inside of the wrist, up to and past the inside of the elbow, and even along the underside of their upper arm. This skin is soft and subtle, but doesn't get much love. It frequently feels incredible. Ditto goes for starting at their ankles and kissing all the way up past the area behind their knees to their thighs. Inside and behind joints (wrists, elbows, knees, ankles) may be particularly sensitive, and even ticklish to touch and kissing—if your partner is super ticklish, you can always move to another area.

The Erogenous Zone's Connected to the Hip Bone

Other areas that might love a little extra attention are the sides of the body, all the way down to and including the hip bones. Again, these areas don't usually get any touch, especially not soft and sensual touch, so it can feel truly incredible to have them gently touched, licked, kissed, and so on.

Get Their Digits

Don't forget the fingers and toes (and the hands and feet to which they're attached). Some people love the idea of gently taking clean fingers (or toes) into their mouth and sucking on them. To some, this is super gross. Still others couldn't care less either way. Figure out where you are, and decide this before you're in the moment.

If you decide to go for it, start out gently. You can always increase pressure, add suction, swirl your tongue around their digits, and so on. Sometimes people like to suck on a finger or lick it in a way that mimics oral sex—it might just be a super-hot way to turn someone on, or it could even be a precursor of things to come (pun oh-so intended). You can also combine massaging hands and feet with orally stimulating them, or choose to just give a nice foot or hand massage. If you decide to go that route, just remember that while some people find hand and foot massages to be sexually arousing and even invigorating, others find them to be wonderfully relaxing ... so relaxing, in fact, that they might fall asleep after your absolutely amazing massage. Of course, there's nothing wrong with this (after all, helping your partner get into such a relaxed and destressed state is an awesome skill to have), but it can be a little disappointing if you're in the mood to get it on, and your lover's in the mood to be counting sheep. Just think ahead.

Anywhere Your Heart (and Loins) Desire

Of course, there are many more areas that can feel wonderful. The small of the back, the scalp (as in a scalp massage—you may not want to lick their hair ... or maybe you do!), the armpits (some people love being that close to the pheromones that get them going), the belly button, and the list goes on. If it's covered in skin, it can enjoy touch. This means pretty much the whole body. Just remember, different people enjoy different types of touch, and in different areas of their body, so experiment and explore to figure out where and how YOU like to be touched, as well as the same information for your partner, and suddenly, a few kisses here and there have turned into a professional turn-on session, and you're golden!

Chapter

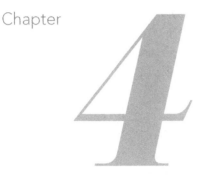

Communication Skills — Tell Me What You REALLY Want

Communication is key. I cannot stress that enough. If you can't communicate with the person with whom you're having sex, then why the heck are you having sex with them? I mean, really?

Now, communication about sex doesn't need to look like sitting down with a negotiation form and having a looooong, drawn-out conversation about each of your sexual histories, all your likes and dislikes, every single need and want, every single turn-off and dislike, health history, and so on (although if that's what works best for you, then absolutely go for it). Sexual communication could look like this, if you were, say, hooking up in a bar or club bathroom:

You: Hey, I'm Jane!

Them: Hey, I'm Taylor!

Jane: I like giving oral sex, receiving oral sex, and being fingered up against the wall.

Taylor: I like giving oral sex and fingering people up against the wall.

Jane: Awesome, why don't you finger fuck me against the wall and go down on me.

Taylor: Sweet. What does safer sex look like for you?

Jane: Here's a glove and a dam.

Taylor: Right on.

See, it doesn't have to be anything too in-depth (pun intended). The very bottom level of sexual communication is what do you each like, what does safer sex look like (with a new person), and perhaps each others' names if you don't happen to know that already. Of course, you can absolutely build on it from there, learning about which spots people like to be kissed on or telling your partner what they can whisper in your ear to make you wet, but it can be just as basic as what you want to do.

Imagine the above scenario. What if there had been NO communication, and Jane just assumed that she should go down on Taylor. Taylor isn't into that, so that could have ended their sexual tryst right there and then. Luckily, they had just enough communication to make sure that they were doing something that both of them enjoyed, and that whatever safer sex they wanted to have happen was actually happening. Ta-da! Isn't communication great?

So now that we have the basic definition of what communication is out of the way, let's get started on how to communicate. We'll be figuring out if you're most comfortable:

X--- Communicating what your needs are using the compliment sandwich, "find my favorite spots," or sexy sticky notes.

X--- Discovering new things using the optometrist style, going back to school, or watching movies for two.

Communicating What Your Needs Are

We don't usually have a lot of skills for communicating sexually, mostly because it was never something we were taught. Not only that, we haven't had a lot of practice, since we've been told that sexual chemistry is supposed to be innate. If things aren't going right, it means that something's wrong with one of you, and it wasn't meant to be … which is bullcrap! So, here are a couple of easy ways to format sexual communication so that it's helpful (not hurtful), fun, and provides good feedback to all involved. You may feel a little awkward at first when talking about sex, but if you're comfortable doing the deed, you can get comfortable talking about it.

Which of these seems like your style?

➤ *The Compliment Sandwich, page 53*

➤ *Find My Favorite Spots, page 54*

➤ *Sexy Sticky Notes, page 56*

❥ *The Compliment Sandwich*

This is an activity (very short, can be done anywhere and at any time) in which you give your partner feedback in a sandwich. The ingredients of said sandwich are specific:

Positive Comment

Suggestion for Change

Positive Comment

All in all, it's a sandwich with the goal of creating some of the change(s) that you'd like to see while making your partner feel good about themselves and the things they're good at. Win-win? Yes!

The two "slices of bread" (the positive comments) should be created out of genuine and wonderful compliments about things that are going right. Use these to help remind your partner of how much you like being with them and how awesome being sexual with them feels to you. Then, the "filling" of the sandwich (the suggestion for change) is a positive (decidedly not passive aggressive) change that you'd like to see happen while sexual activity is taking place. This gives you the opportunity to give them feel-good feedback, as well as feedback that requires action or change of some sort, all while making an effort to not end up with hurt feelings on either side. Here are two examples:

Example #1:

Wow! You look amazing when you're down there between my legs!

I wish you'd go down on me for like twenty minutes.

I am so turned on by you eating me out!

Example #2:

I love it when you take me from behind, because it feels so good!

Mmm … if you could rub my clit/use a vibe on my clit while you do it …

I bet I could come like five times because you're so good at it.

The "filling" layer (the change you'd like to happen) can be feedback on anything, including timing, positions, pressure, reactions (or lack thereof), and so forth. Regardless of what it is that you need, try using the compliment sandwich to get the message across while still giving your partner some great feedback about how much you enjoy being sexual with them.

As a side note, the compliment sandwich can improve communications in relationships outside just sexual interactions. Consider using it to get more time together (or less time together!), to make sure chores are done, or to talk about subjects that might otherwise feel that you're just nagging your partner, which might result in a fight or passive aggression.

Example:

You're so supportive of my busy schedule, and I appreciate it!

Do you think you could have dinner on the table when I get home?

Your lasagna is absolutely to die for, and I'm really craving it.

➤ *Find My Favorite Spots*

Communication doesn't have to mean exchanging words. Another fun game that embodies communication (albeit in a less than verbal way) is called "find my favorite spots." Perhaps you and your partner are new to exploring each other's bodies, or maybe you've been together for a long time and feel that you're in a sexual rut. This is a great way to help them discover some of your spots that could use a bit more attention and/or stimulation … and you can always switch it up and have them do it for you.

Step 1: Figure out something that your partner finds tasty. Traditionally, people use honey dust or just plain honey, but you could use chocolate, BBQ sauce, or whatever is orally motivating for them. (Note: Do not put anything containing sugar on/near your vulva. You're just asking for a yeast infection.)

Step 2: Send your partner out of the room, and choose between three and five erogenous zones, or spots that you want them to find and stimulate. Put a dab of whatever you decided in step one on each spot — not too much because that makes it too obvious.

Step 3: Call your partner back. Either with or without a blindfold (depending on how difficult you want it to be), ask them to find the spots with their mouth, and their mouth only. You can tell them how many there are, or just make them keep going until they've discovered all the spots. This is a great chance to get them to focus on sensitive areas other than just your genitals, since they have to actively explore your body to find your sweet spots. Another option for people who are more olfactory motivated (i.e., scent gets them going a lot more than taste) is to dab on your favorite perfume or essential oil, and then blindfold them and ask them to find it using only their nose.

Once they've found your spots, you can discuss what you'd like them to do to said spots. For some, you might prefer licking, biting, or sucking, while others you might just want them to stroke it or gently slide their nails down it. This way, not only do they have a better idea of WHERE you'd like to be touched, but also

HOW you'd like to be stimulated in each of these areas. Again, feel free to switch it up so that they can share their spots with you as well!

❥ *Sexy Sticky Notes*

Unless you have an office supply fetish, sticky notes might not be what gets you going. However, there are ways that you can use them to help communicate your sexual wants and needs to your partner.

Suggestion A

Buy or borrow (you'd be surprised at the number of sexuality books you can borrow at your local library—holy cow!) a book on sex. It can be something general like *The Guide to Getting It On*, or something on a specific topic (like *Oral Sex That'll Blow Her Mind*), or just use this book, and use sticky notes to flag some of the pages that have activities or ideas that interest you. You can write on them or just leave them blank—whichever works best with your communication style. Then, leave the book on your partner's nightstand, or hide it in their backpack or briefcase (probably not before a huge meeting, because that could be more stressful to them than helpful).

When you see them next (or after a certain amount of time that feels good to you, like a day, a week, or a month), casually bring up the book and the sticky notes. "Hey, what did you think about those marked pages? Does that seem like something that you'd like to try, or that you think we could try?" You don't have to start the conversation from square one, and it gives them time to read about it, think about the idea, and come up with how they'll react to you. Of course, they may not like it at all, but instead of getting a screwed-up face and saying, "EWWWW—GROSS!"

because they were caught off guard, they might just say, "You know what, that isn't really my thing, but hey, maybe we can try _____" because they had time to think.

On the other hand, maybe they were hoping to try that exact same thing too, but didn't know how to bring it up in conversation with you. Now you both know you're into it and can either discuss how to make it happen or even just go ahead and make it happen. Heck, you might not even get a chance to discuss the sticky notes; it's always possible that they'll take the hint and move forward with the idea without waiting for a discussion.

Suggestion B

Another option you have with sticky notes is to write things on them (so avant-garde, I know) and position them around the house/apartment/hotel room. If you want there to be more temperature play, you could leave a note on the freezer that says something to the effect of, "I know a place or two you could put these ice cubes …" or, even more direct, "Bring these to the bedroom." You can be roundabout or specific, whatever works for you and your relationship and/or communication style.

Want sex in the shower? A note like "We could really make things steamy in here" or "All this shower needs is two hot bodies" can let your partner know about your intents. You can also get more creative. Want some spanking with a hairbrush? Leave a note on their hairbrush saying, "I bet this brush would like to see some action!" Or want to tell them that you're ready for some sexual interactions (regardless of what they might be)? A note with something to the effect of "Looks like this won't be seeing any ZZZs tonight!" on their pillow is a great way to let them know you'd like things other than sleep to go down in bed tonight.

Options Unlimited

There are lots of ways you can use sticky notes. Put them on the mirror to tell them how sexy you think they are. Put one on some hot underwear that you'd like them to wear on your date out that night. Leave one on their nightstand if you don't live together, letting them know that you'd definitely like to be doing this (or some of the things that you enjoyed this time around) again. You could even leave one on a near-empty bottle of lube that says "Fill me—you'll be needing it!" to remind them to get a new bottle of lube before your next sexual encounter. Not only can it be fun and exciting to create a trail of sticky notes, almost like a treasure map, but it can be a great way to communicate with someone who might not be as verbal or who might get embarrassed at having to sit down and talk about sex. Whatever way you decide to use sticky notes, enjoy and go to town!

Discovering New Things

So you've figured out some basic communication skills. You know how to compliment your partner while also getting your needs met, or how to mark things that you might want to discuss or try later. What about figuring out how to discover the sexual things that each of you likes when you're in the bedroom, getting it on?

Here are some approaches that might make things much more satisfying for you beneath the covers. Which of the following sounds the most appealing?

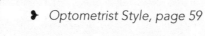

❥ *Optometrist Style*

You know when you go to the optometrist, and the doc gives you different options and asks, "Which is better, number 1 or number 2? Number 2 or number 3?" Yep, that. You're going to try it during sex.

Number 1 or Number 2?

This may seem a little silly to you, and you and your partner may need a bit of a sense of humor to pull it off, but it's a good tool for calibrating your sexy times. Think about starting with something easy. Maybe nibble on your partner's ear one way, and then the other. You can either fully commit to the optometrist style and literally ask them which one they prefer more, number 1 or number 2, OR you can be more suave and ask which feels better, which is hotter, which turns them on more. The same goes for licks, strokes, bites, motions — you name it.

Precision Feedback without the Prickliness

We can often have a difficult time telling someone exactly what it is we want sexually (heck, half the time WE don't even know what feels good, much less how to describe it and explain it to someone else!). However, if someone does something to us, and we're given the immediate opportunity to provide feedback, we can gain a much better grasp of what we like and what doesn't feel as good. Plus, it's a nice way to solicit feedback in a way that doesn't feel like you're asking them for a point-to-point tour of their body, and it gives them the option of letting you know how things are going without feeling like they might offend you.

❥ *Back to School*

Are you with a new partner, or is your longtime partner missing your hot spots? Never fear; here's a tried-and-true way to educate your partner about what feels good and what types of touch, licks, and other sensations you like to receive.

Hot for Teacher

For this, it's time for you to become the teacher. If you're into some hot role-play, you might put on a teacher-like outfit or ask your oh-so-willing student to put on a school tie or plaid skirt. Otherwise, you can do it wearing whatever you want (including nothing) and set the scene verbally.

First, let them know that you'll be providing a class/workshop/lecture today, and the subject is "My Turn-Ons" or "[your name here]'s Body 101"—feel free to get creative and come up with a title that works for you. If you want, you can have them sit in a chair and maybe even tie them there if you feel that they might try to get a little hands-on before you're ready to let them do the practicum.

Hands-on Teaching Skills

Step back, and begin your lesson. If they usually rip off your clothes and you want it to be more sensual, start with a bit of a striptease to slowly show them how you like your shirt unbuttoned just one button at a time (or vice versa—if they're being all kinds of romantic, and you want to show them that all you need is your pants around your ankles, then this is the time).

Take your time to show how and where you like to be touched on your neck, ears, face, and elsewhere. You can choose to either just show or add some adjectives: "I like it when you suck gently on my neck here" or "I love rough nibbling on my ear lobes." For some things, like kissing, you could tell them to relax their lips and say that you're going to show them exactly how you like to be kissed, and then kiss them.

As you move down your body and get into the nether regions, you can go as far as you want. If you like having toys used on you, then show off—what settings, how fast, how hard you want them used, and so forth. You can put on a whole show by yourself, or you can invite them to try out what they've learned. You can even put your hand on top of theirs as they stroke you, showing them what type of pressure you want used and how fast you want them to go.

Final Marks

If you're feeling into it, give feedback as it goes, or even make a fun (and sexy) report card for them at the end. Make sure to emphasize the things they did really well (positive reinforcement can go a looooong way!), and add just a few things they might need to do over and over again in detention. You can take this as far as you want, especially if you decide to make classroom time a regular thing!

❧ *Movies for Two*

A lot of people feel that porn is not designed for couples and that it's a one-person show. However, lots of couples enjoy watching adult movies together. For more of an overview on how to use porn to get things going, turn to the chapter on stimulating your senses. To use movies as an educational tool, read on.

Porno-U

For this topic, I'm talking about educational adult movies. Porn with a purpose, that is. There are many types of educational porn out there, for both singles and couples to increase their knowledge of sex as a whole, and more specifically on certain activities. These videos are fun and tasteful, and many are written, directed, and even hosted by sex educators who know their stuff.

Vivid-Ed is a great line of educational porn and features educators like Tristan Taormino. Adam & Eve education videos feature folks like Nina Hartley, a porn star and registered nurse. The Pleasure Ed series from Good Vibrations stars Dr. Carol Queen, a well-known sexologist and lover of pleasure. All these types of films showcase sex educators, sexologists, and other purveyors of pleasure discussing various types of sex (think oral, anal, G-spot, kink, threesomes, double penetration, etc.), and then have hot porn stars to demonstrate what you just learned.

Watch and Learn

If you and your partner are interested in checking out a new type of sexual activity, or even just taking it to another level with additional information and skills, these movies are great. You can watch them together, talk about what you want to try, and then practice what you just learned; or you can each watch them on your own, pick up some new tricks to wow your partner, and show off the next time you get it on.

The nice thing about these videos is that not only are you getting good, accurate information that can help you understand what's going on with your body (and your partner's body), but you're also getting some nice eye candy for visual stimulation that demonstrates the type of sex you want, done in a way that shows off authentic pleasure. A win-win all around!

Chapter

Orgasmic Bliss – Info about Orgasms

Everyone loves to talk about orgasms. Are you having them? How many are you having? What do they feel like? How intense are yours?

Orgasms are more than just the fabulous exploding feeling of pleasure that's located in a certain area or that goes throughout your body. In fact, a huge body of research has been done on orgasms. While some people might think that science is not the sexiest subject, learning about your own body and how it responds to sexual stimulation is fascinating and can help you to have a more fulfilling sex life. That's why this chapter will be exploring:

X--- The journey of an orgasm from excitement to plateau to pleasure and finally recovery, as described in the research of Bill Masters and Virginia Johnson.

X--- Multiple orgasms: What are some ways to try to get from one to tons?

The Journey of an Orgasm

The research duo of Bill Masters and Virginia Johnson helped developed a theory of the human sexual response cycle. This four-stage model shows how your body responds physiologically while you're being sexually stimulated. These four stages are the excitement phase, the plateau phase, the orgasmic phase, and the resolution phase. Folks of all sexes and genders go through these phases during sex (although some might just go through excitement and plateau without hitting orgasm, or they may be able to go through the first three stages multiple times without much time, or any at all, in the resolution phase).

Now that you know about the different phases of the human sexual response cycle, which one do you want to learn more about first?

➤ *The Excitement Phase, page 66*

➤ *The Plateau Phase, page 69*

➤ *The Pleasure Phase, page 69*

➤ *The Recovery Phase, page 70*

❥ *The Excitement Phase*

The excitement phase is the gateway to arousal. When you enter this phase, it's usually because something caused you to start feeling turned on. It could have been a sensual or sexual thought, some kissing, some groping, or dirty words being whispered in your ear. If it gets your motor going, it's beginning the excitement phase.

What Does This Look Like for Your Body?

Your heartbeat starts to speed up, as does your respiration. Your blood pressure starts to rise. In this situation, that's OK; in fact, it's a good thing. Many women experience something called the "sex flush," which is a reddening or blushing of the chest and back. This rise in color is even on some people and blotchy on others. Your nipples probably become erect (although not always), and your breasts may start swelling slightly as they begin to feel more sensual and reactive to touch.

This is when most women begin the lubrication process, although it's important to remember that not all women lubricate or lubricate a large amount, and that lubrication is not always an indication of arousal. Also, your vaginal muscles may start to tighten and your uterus will start to pull back into your body (you probably can't feel this), creating more space in the vaginal canal. And, oh yeah, blood starts rushing into your genitals, making your clitoris and labia swell, which can be a pretty pleasant sensation.

What Do You Do with All This Excitement?

As far as what to do while you're in the excitement period, the answer is whatever feels good to you. Your genitals may feel ready for direct touch or stimulation, or you may feel that you need a lot more stimulation before you're ready for hands-on.

The excitement phase can last anywhere from just a few minutes to a few hours, and you can spend that time watching porn, having sexy thoughts read aloud to you, making out, having your partner run their hands all over your body, or even having them lick, stroke, suck, or otherwise stimulate your vulva. Each woman and her body are totally different, so get in tune with yours so you can ask for what you need.

❥ *The Plateau Phase*

The plateau phase is the second of the four phases of the human sexual response cycle and not nearly as boring as it sounds. It follows the excitement phase and involves more physiological changes in your body. It's the excitement phase squared: you'll experience increased respiration, your heart beating even faster than it was before, your blood pressure continuing to rise. This is when the clitoris, which was coaxed out via stimulation and vasocongestion (blood rushing to the genitals) in the excitement phase, may become increasingly sensitive and may actually pull back in under the hood (which can be incredibly frustrating to both you and your partner alike!). Your labia and vagina will continue to swell as more blood comes to your genital region, and if you're someone who lubricates a fair amount, this may be where lubrication really starts flowing.

Usually you get to this stage of the response cycle when your entire vulva (labia, mons pubis, clitoris, clitoral hood) is being stimulated by a tongue, lips, fingers, a sexy toy, and you may be experiencing some penetration as well, of fingers, a penis, or a dildo. This stage is pleasurable by itself, but it usually leads into an even more pleasurable state of being, known as the pleasure phase, which is the phase in which orgasm or climax takes place.

Ready to Launch

The plateau phase usually happens right before an orgasm for most people, although in women who have yet to have an orgasm, this can be incredibly satisfying by itself. That being said, sometimes if you and your body are kept at this stage too long, it can feel frustrating, similar to men getting "blue balls." Just like blue balls, you can alleviate the frustration or pressure by masturbating yourself to orgasm if you're unable to climax with your partner. While it can feel frustrating, it's certainly not dangerous to your body or your mind to be continually stimulated in the plateau phase and not achieve orgasm.

Failure to Launch

Are you among the large number of women unable to orgasm? Not to worry! Lots of ladies are in this situation, but you can likely get out of it with a little dedication. The first thing to consider is whether you're able to orgasm on your own. If so, the rest of this book can provide suggestions on how to communicate with your partner about your needs. If you're not able to orgasm on your own, and have tried things like vibrators (if you haven't, DEFINITELY try vibrators), then I'd suggest that you chat with your gynecologist to rule out medical issues. Around 20 percent of women in the United States have some sort of vulvar pain disorder at some point in their life, and this can impede orgasms, as can imbalances of some hormones.

If everything checks out hunky-dory, try exploring the different things that turn you on (erotica, porn, dirty talk, scents, etc.), and pair them with masturbation. Bring yourself to arousal and then back off. Don't start with the ultimate goal of an orgasm; aim for experiencing a variety of sexual pleasure. The more you focus on having an elusive orgasm, the more stressed out you'll be and the less likely it is that you'll be successful. Explore other ways to experience pleasure, like breasts/nipple stimulation, spankings, anal stimulation, and practice redefining your views of orgasms and sexual pleasure.

❥ *The Pleasure Phase*

The pleasure phase is the third phase of the four-stage human sexual response cycle. When people think of sexual response and pleasure, this is the stage that they most often picture, in which orgasm and/or climax happens. When you have an orgasm, your heart rate continues to increase as it has through the previous two stages. Your pelvic floor muscles contract (and you can also experience contractions of your uterus and vagina), and you'll likely feel extreme pleasure. Depending on the type of stimulation and the type of orgasm, as well as your individual body, you may feel pleasure located specifically in the genitals, or as waves crashing over your body, at the base of your spine, from the tips of your fingers to the tips of your toes, and in all sorts of other ways. If you asked ten different women to describe their orgasms, they would likely all have different descriptions and might even have different answers for different types of orgasms that they have from different stimulation. When you climax, your other muscles may contract involuntarily, and you may also experience gasping, moaning, shouting, screaming, or other involuntary sounds coming from your mouth.

Making the Most of It

As far as what to do while you're in the pleasure stage, it depends completely on your body and what feels good. Some women enjoy continued penetration during climax, while others prefer for the inserted object to be removed while they're having their orgasm. You may like clitoral and vulvar stimulation even after you've completed your climax, or you may want it to stop immediately because you've become incredibly sensitive to sensations. Again, everyone is completely different, and you can experiment until you find out what works best for you. Once you do, make sure you communicate those tricks and techniques that work best on your body to your partner (or partners), so that they can help provide the best possible orgasmic experiences for you. After your orgasm (or orgasms!), your body moves into the recovery stage.

❯ *The Recovery Phase*

The recovery phase is the fourth and final phase of the four-stage human sexual response cycle. It occurs after you've completed the pleasure phase, which usually involves one or more orgasms. Your blood pressure decreases, and your heart rate and respiration start to slow down, heading back toward normal. Your muscles, which may have been contracted during orgasm, are given the opportunity to relax and unclench.

Ready for Round Two?

The time between climaxing and being able to start the sexual response cycle again is frequently known as the "refractory period." Given this, while men almost all have refractory periods of at least a minute or two (and up to a few hours), many women have an incredibly short refractory period, or absolutely none at all, and can continue to receive stimulation starting immediately after their orgasm, allowing them to have multiple and extended orgasms. Other women may find that their clitoris is incredibly sensitive after climax, and it may even hurt or feel uncomfortable to have it touched. In those cases, continued stimulation of the breasts, nipples, thighs, labia, and other parts can help bring you back to the excitement or even plateau phase, moving comfortably toward another orgasm.

Multiple Orgasms

Now that we've covered the basics about orgasms, how they happen, and the phases of the human sexual response cycle, it's time to talk about multiple orgasms. Are they real? Can everyone have multiple orgasms? What defines a multiple orgasm? How do I know whether I'm having multiples?

All these questions help add mystery and mystique around multiple orgasms. The answer to "Can everyone have multiples?" is likely yes, though not everyone has figured out how to do so or can do so with any specific type of sexual stimulation. Not everyone even wants to have multiple orgasms. It can be tricky to know whether you're having multiples. For some people, they are very distinct orgasms—they actually go back through the whole sexual response cycle, including resolution, and just start the process over again, albeit very quickly. Other people might feel that they're having only one orgasm, but it lasts two or three minutes and might be made up of dozens of little orgasms, all happening back to back to back. As I've discussed already, there's no holy grail in sex, and that includes having multiple orgasms.

The question I pose is why does it matter whether you're having multiples, as long as you're enjoying yourself? Lots of people are hungry for more information on having just one or more than one orgasm. To find out more, pick where you're at right now for number of orgasms:

➤ *One Is Fun! page 72*

➤ *Give Me More ... page 73*

➤ *I Just Can't Get Enough! page 75*

➤ *One Is Fun!*

For now at least, you're a one-orgasm kind of gal. You like to work your way through the phases of the sexual response cycle, and when you finally get to the climax, you give it all that you have. What you need to think about is whether that's enough for you. Many women enjoy having one orgasm at a time, and that works out perfectly for them. If you're happy with what's going on, keep reading. Otherwise, head down to the "Give Me More ..." section.

The Big One

While one orgasm might not seem as gratifying as having two or ten or more, if you make it count, and find it sexually satisfying, then that's what matters. You can play around with getting orgasms from different types of stimulation. For many people, an orgasm derived mostly from clitoral stimulation is going to feel much different than an orgasm that comes predominantly from vaginal stimulation, and if you have both types of stimulation at the same time, you might even find another type of feeling when you climax. You can also add other sensations like anal stimulation, being spanked, wearing nipple clamps, and so on, which can change the way that your body experiences orgasms.

Ditto with mixing up the senses. Wearing a blindfold while you climax is going to enhance all your other senses, really changing up the whole orgasm experience for you.

It's YOUR Orgasm

Sadly, some people get a bit judgmental about how different types of people have sex, and you might run into some preachy folks who say that you can never be truly sexually satisfied having only one orgasm at a time. To that, I call bullshit. If you're doing what feels good and fulfilling to you, and you're happy with your sex life, then don't let anyone else and their idea of what a "good sex life" or "sexually satisfied woman" looks like make you question yourself or change any of your habits. Do what feels good, and you're set for life!

❥ *Give Me More …*

You want more, more, more and want to know how to have multiples. While many people believe that all women are capable of achieving multiple orgasms, it's also true that many women have tried and have not yet been able to figure out how to make that happen. So make sure as you explore the wonderful world of multiple orgasms in a row that you don't put too much emphasis on succeeding. As long as you enjoy the sex that you're having, you're good to go. Obsessing over something like not being able to have multiple orgasms can cause issues in the bedroom rather than elevate your sex life.

Don't Stop Till You've Had Enough

So, the next time that you're either masturbating or having someone get you off by oral sex, manual stimulation, or a vibrator, ask them to keep on providing the sensation after you've already climaxed. It may feel intense at first to continue the sensation (and you may want to dial down the speed on the vibe or tell them to slow down with the intensity of their licking), but take some deep breaths through it. It can help to push out with your Kegel muscles: that may feel slightly less intense for your body. Continue to enjoy the sensation, and eventually you may start to feel your body ramping up again. If you do, just let your body do its thing.

Take a Breather

You may not be able to have multiple orgasms by continuing stimulation; some women do have that refractory period and need a few minutes of no stimulation before it'll feel good to be stimulated again. If that's you, take a break. You can make out, have your partner play with your nipples, run their nails down your back, and so on. Once you start feeling turned on again (as compared to still recovering from your last orgasm), let them resume the genital stimulation. You may feel that the second, third, and other additional orgasms are more or less intense than your first, or they might be completely different. Multiple orgasms are still multiples if they happen in the same sexy session, regardless of how you reach them and whether you need a break in between.

Don't Let Frustration Ruin a Good Time

If you're not having much success in getting multiples to happen, take a break. Sometimes, we put waaaay too much pressure on making something work that just isn't going to happen at all. Ditto goes for if your partner has some "goal" of "making" you have multiple orgasms. If you set specific goals for sexual activity, rather than just aiming to enjoy yourselves and have fun, you're setting the bar pretty high, which makes not reaching it feel that much more frustrating. Don't let anyone tell you that you have to or even should learn how to have multiple orgasms. Do it at your own pace, and you'll get there if and when it's time.

❥ *I Just Can't Get Enough!*

You're already queen of multiple orgasms and enjoy riding the waves of your climax like there's no tomorrow. Whether you have your multiples back to back to back, or with a few moments of downtime in between, you know how to make your body sing, and you're able to communicate your wants and needs to your partner. Good for you! If you're happy with where you are and how things are going, why work to change a good thing? You never know, you might stumble on an even better way to have orgasms. So experiment, and try some new things to improve or even just diversify your multiple orgasm experiences.

New Frontiers

Consider moving beyond what's tried-and-true and adding in new elements. If you always tend to climax in the same position, try seeing if you can achieve satisfaction in a different position, which may lead to a different orgasm. Always reach your orgasms in the same way? Since you know that you can definitely make it work, try other types of stimulation (clitoral, penetrative, clitoral, and penetrative, climaxing with penetration at the same time, climaxing while having the penetrative object pulled out of you). Experiment with various sex toys to see whether different vibrators change the sensation, or if wearing a butt plug (or receiving other types of anal stimulation) makes your orgasms better or at least different. Maybe do some kinky power play where you work on delaying your orgasms over and over so that they're that much more intense once you finally have them. There are lots of ways to mix things up in the world of orgasms.

Own It!

Also, please don't ever feel ashamed about your ability to have multiple orgasms. It comes easily (pun is oh-so intended) to some people, and may be difficult to figure out for others. Everyone is their own person, and your ability to come and come and come is something that makes you special and unique in your own way. Own and love it, and keep coming till the cows come home!

6

Stimulating the Senses

There's so much more to sex than just putting Tab A into, onto, or next to Slot B. In fact, while some folks may be able to go from 0 to 60 in 3.5 seconds, many other folks need to have their senses stimulated in various ways. This could include hearing sexy things, looking at sensual things, sharing a hot conversation with one another, or any other types of ways to stimulate these senses.

In this chapter, you're going to discover:

X--- What stimulates your mind? Erotica read aloud, watching hot and heavy movies, or sexting with your sweet thing?

X--- Super-sensation play! When it comes to touch, what gets you tingling: something soft and fuzzy, hot and cold, or sharp and scratchy?

What Stimulates Your Mind?

First, let's talk about which of the following appeals to you the most when it comes to stimulating the senses and getting your imagination revving. Which of these seems like it would get you going the most?

▶ *Reading Erotica, page 78*

▶ *Watching Hot and Heavy Porn, page 81*

▶ *Sending Salacious Texts and E-mails, page 86*

Of those options, choose the one that's going to help you arouse all those things that make up your sexual senses.

▶ *Reading Erotica*

Sounds like you're into auditory stimulation, which means you like to hear things, and process them that way. Using some super-sensual erotica is a great way to get down and dirty in the arousal department. How you choose the right erotica can be a bit more of a challenge.

There are as many types of erotica out there as there are types of sex and sexual activity. Into romance novels? There's erotica for that. More into female dominance? They've got erotica for that. All about lesbian lovers getting it on? You can find erotica for that. So the first step to figuring out the right kind of erotica to bring into the bedroom (or wherever you'll be reading it!) is to identify what you're looking for.

The Erotica That's Right for You

If you want something more delicately phrased that uses wording like "his sword sheathed in velvet" and "her flowery lotus," then look for romance novels with buff guys and busty women on the cover, and fast-forward to the sex scenes. While most romance novels, especially the ones available at bookstores and the grocery, feature heterosexual male-female couples, you can definitely find ones featuring two women. They make ones that are historical, if you're into it taking two to tango on the Titanic, or getting it on during the *Gone with the Wind* era, or you can find more modern books featuring the mattress mambo.

On the other hand, if you just want sex, sex, sex, and nothing else, check out some of the erotica that features sexy short stories; quickies for the mind, basically. There are many available for purchase online and even in most bookstores; an example is *Got A Minute? 60-Second Erotica*. Some of these books have tons of hot stories that are fewer than two thousand words—that means that you don't have to wait long before the sex starts, and it only gets more delicious from there. Most of these stories aren't going to have specific themes, but are just balls to the wall (pun totally intended) sex.

More in the middle? Look for one of the hundreds of erotica anthologies that exist. Most have a theme; some are based more on the quality of the work, like each year's compilation of *Best Women's Erotica*, while others can be very specific. *Cheeky Spanking Stories* is about just that, while *Wetter: True Lesbian Sex Stories* is also pretty self-explanatory. *Duty and Desire* is a bunch of yummy stories about members of the military, while *Take Me There* features transgender and genderqueer folks in the vignettes.

Story Time

So you've figured out what book is the best fit for you and your partner—now what? You have two options: the first is to skim through the book(s) in advance (or they can do it without you seeing) and choose a story or scene that turns you on. Cuddle up with your loved one, and slowly, sensually, read out the story. Another choice is to just stick your finger into the middle of the book and start reading (or go to the beginning of that story or sex scene). It's kind of like erotica roulette, and you both know that you'll be at least somewhat surprised with what you get. You may feel a little silly at first, but push through and give it an earnest try. Once you get into it, the rewards are stellar.

You could stop with just one, and head to the bed, or couch, or kitchen table, to act it out, or turn to another story to keep the foreplay going. If you're into delayed gratification, consider reading stories out loud to each other before you go on a date, or have your partner drive and read something scrumptious to them on the way to dinner and a movie. You'll both be all kinds of turned on, and be forced to wait just a bit longer to rip off each other's clothes. Not into paper books? Good news! Most erotica is available in eBook formats, so download now for a good time later.

The Golden Age of the Internet

Not ready to purchase an entire anthology of erotica yet? Good news! The Internet is good for porn ... including the written stuff. Sites like LitErotica.com let a bevy of users submit their own creations, and again, you can find erotica on pretty much every topic you could imagine, and probably some that you can't. Plus, there are thousands of sex bloggers out there, writing in dirty detail about their devious sexual exploits. Put some key words in the search engine of your choice and voilà; all the erotica you could want. You can even access it on your smartphones and tablets, for sensual erotica on the go.

The U in Author

If you want to take it a step further, consider writing your own erotica. A great place to start is retelling some of the steamiest sex you've already had. Perhaps it's already playing on repeat from a movie reel in your head, or you masturbate to it as you relive all the fabulous things that happened. Why not turn it into your own story for posterity, and use it to ready yourself and your partner to get down and dirty all over again? Sit in front of the computer—or you can handwrite it in a journal if you prefer—and start listing the highlights. What were each of you wearing? Who touched whom? Where did they get touched? Add a few adjectives, fill in the blanks, and BAM! You have custom-made erotica based on your real-life amazing sexcapades. Some of the benefits: you know it's going to turn you on, it uses the same language for body parts that you do, and you know that you can absolutely visualize those foxy folks getting it on.

Whatever way you decide to rock the erotica, open your ears and get ready for some deliciously delectable foreplay.

❥ *Watching Hot and Heavy Porn*

Many people seem to have the erroneous idea that porn is all a man's game and that it's designed to never cross the threshold of a woman's home, or *gasp* find its way into a couple's bedroom. I'm happy to be able to tell you that this is in fact not the case. The world of porn is not only open to women; there are female directors, porn "geared" to women and couples, queer porn, gay porn, porn with plots, porn with absolutely no plots, porn parodies, porn vignettes, niche porn on every possible subject you could imagine, porn made on the sets of mainstream movies, and much more. This is a real-life enactment of the idea that "if you build it, they will come." There's enough porn out there to turn on anyone of any orientation, gender, age (over eighteen, of course), and sexual inclination.

Why Do People Watch Porn?

For a myriad of reasons. Lots of people are stimulated by visual or auditory things, and a good porno can provide both. Whether naked bodies banging together gets your motor revving, or the sensuous sounds of one, two, or more people is what brings your blood to a boil, porn is great way to sit down with your partner and exponentially increase the horniness factor in a flash.

I'm not saying that porn is for everyone; what I am saying is don't knock it based on what you may have heard. If you've tried a few different adult video/DVD/streaming options and you're still not feeling it, that's absolutely OK, too. It's just one more item to try from the smorgasbord, and if it turns out that it isn't your cup of tea (or your screenshot of hot, sweaty bodies), then move on to your next sexploration.

Pick Your Porn Provider

But if you do get a little tingle at the site of some skin on screen, let's talk about choosing porn. There are so many choices out there that it can feel overwhelming. First, you need to figure out how you'd like to partake in said porn. If you have a laptop and can stream dirty movies online, there are loads of places to find porn. While some are free, I'd highly suggest trying the paid stuff; not only are you supporting the performers, directors, and crew by purchasing their work, you're also going to get better quality.

A great place to start is the website HotMoviesForHer.com. Run by women, this site has tens of thousands of films to watch, and you pay by the minute, which is awesome. This means that rather than buy a movie that you might not like, you can buy, say, one hundred, five hundred, or even one thousand minutes and spend them watching various scenes from favorite producers featuring favorite stars, so you can get an idea of what turns you on, what makes you laugh, and what you might just find boring. They have films geared to all orientations, but offer significantly more hetero films, given the industry.

If you're looking for some hot queer porn to stream online, CrashPadSeries.com is one of the longest-running, sexiest queer porn sites out there, and QueerPorn.tv is a newer yet super-fulfilling site offering queer porn of all persuasions.

Into more kinky stuff? FetishMovies.com is more video on demand, and the family of Kink.com sites (MenInPain.com, Hogtied.com, FuckingMachines.com, and more) offers sexy pictures and video, as well as live shows. PaddedKink.com is specifically for curve-loving kinksters. BurningAngel.com has clips of more alternative folks (think tattoos, piercings, fun colors of hair, etc.) doing the nasty.

Hardcopy Porn

More into the DVD setup? Not a problem! Lots of companies still release thousands of DVDs a year, and there are several awesome smaller, more independent productions. The big names include Digital Playground, Wicked, Adam & Eve, Vivid, Evil Angel, Pink Visual, Shane's World, Ninn Worx, Jules Jordan, Elegant Angel, New Sensations, and more. You can find titles from most of these studios at almost any adult shop or website. While there are some exceptions, these films are going to feature more of the stereotypical porn—blonde, slim, buxom babes going at it, mostly with super-chiseled men. If that's what gets you going, then for goodness' sake, go for it! However, if you're looking for something a little more specific, unique, realistic, different, there are plenty of options.

Porn with a Plot (and Maybe a Pun)

For hetero films (i.e., men and women getting it on), there are some that have more of a plot. While a few are produced by the studios listed above (like the Pirates porn series, and many of the popular parodies, like *Glee XXX* and *This Ain't the Brady Bunch XXX*, and the list goes on), other studios specialize in porn with a plot. Femme Productions, run by the fabulous Candida Royalle, features couples who look more realistic and offers a lot more in the plot department (although some of these are a bit out-of-date). Comstock Films creates the pornumentary in which you learn about real-life couples, how they met, and how they like to have sex … and then you watch them doing just that. HeartCore productions, distributed by Good Vibrations, has a selection of films that use incredibly sexy performers, have a pretty good semblance of a plot, and showcase authentic pleasure—no faked orgasms in these movies! Sweet Sinner and its lesbian offshoot, Sweetheart Video, both provide plots and real climaxes, featuring both traditional porn stars and those outside what you might expect.

If Hetero Is a No-Go

Looking for something a little less in the binary? Pink and White is a queer production company that features queer and transgender stars getting it on, sometimes with a plot, sometimes without, but always in ways that the performers enjoy, so be ready for lots of hot moans and screams. Trouble Films distributes not only movies from owner Courtney Trouble but also queer porn pioneers like Tobi Hill-Meyer. Early to Bed, a feminist-owned, sex positive toy store in Chicago, filmed their own porn movie, and Delores Park Studios has one or two great queer movies out as well. Good Vibrations also distributes Reel Queer Films, which feature both full-length productions (complete with a plot and lots of sex scenes) and compilations of vignettes that offer real queer folks doing what they love sexually.

Want Something a Little More Educational?

Check out Vivid-Ed's series of educational videos, most of which feature the amazing sex educator Tristan Taormino. Unlike what some people might expect, these films have excellent advice on anal sex, fellatio, cunnilingus, kink, threesomes, and more, followed by some jaw-dropping performances by porn stars, putting what you just learned into action. Nina Hartley also stars in her fair share of educational videos. As a registered nurse and porn star with over four hundred titles to her name, she offers a combination that is fun, sexy, and educational. More recently, Good Vibrations started distributing a sex education line called Pleasure Ed. Currently, they have only a few titles out, but they're fantastic, and great to watch either on your own for education or with a partner to spice things up.

A Good Investment

If you can't find the DVDs that you're looking for in a store, plenty of online sites sell them. Few stores offer rentals anymore, so buying the DVD might be a bit of an investment. Of course, if you find a performer who makes you feel good between your legs, or a studio whose production quality, plots, or bad puns make watching porn an absolute treat, then buy away. Having porn for a rainy day (or really, for whenever you might want to enjoy some of that visual stimulation) is a great investment.

Porn for Pairs

Whatever porn you pick, it's worth chatting with your partner about what you're watching. Remember that what happens in porn isn't always how it goes down (pun intended) in the real world. While you might get ideas from your favorite porn that you want to try out, it's also OK to know that you don't have to try five or six different positions every time you want to get it on.

Don't forget that a lot of things are cut out of porn, like lube application, negotiation, and of course, the silly stuff like people farting, falling off the bed, and so on. The porn that you watch can make for a great fantasy and way to turn you and your lover on, but make sure that you both know that it isn't realistic to emulate porn exactly in your real-life experiences. It just isn't feasible and could lead to some disappointment.

❥ *Sending Salacious Texts and E-mails*

Back in the day (as in pre-twentieth century), love letters were written in beautiful handwriting on paper, sealed with a kiss, and sent through various methods to lovers both near and far. While that idea remains poignant for some (and others might yearn for their loved ones to put down some of their more romantic feelings on actual paper), our technology has changed. While yes, one CAN write a love letter via e-mail, it seems that this world of technological instant gratification has developed many more sexual avenues. Whether you're using Skype, some form of instant messenger (IMing), or just texting on your smartphone, there's now a myriad of ways to reach your partner to tell them exactly what you want to do to them and what kind of action you might be seeking from them in return.

Spell It Out for Me

When pagers first came out, it was a fun challenge for folks to send dirty messages on them, from 696969 to 80085 (which kinda sorta spells "boobs" if you squint your eyes and reach a little). However, with the way technology has advanced in just a few years, we're no longer limited to such archaic pervy messages. Instead, people have come up with their own abbreviations to make sexting (sexy text messaging) more exact, but still hard to understand for the uninitiated. DTF? Down to fuck. IF/IB? In front or in back. IWSN? I Want Sex NOW. TDTM? Talk dirty to me. JEOMK? Just ejaculated on my keyboard (note: you might want to find another place to do that—most computer warranties don't cover ejaculate between the keys). The list goes on.

Sample Sexting Scripts

Confused yet? Don't worry! You don't need to be the mistress of text abbreviations to be DTF technologically with your sweetie. You can send messages (via text, IM, or e-mail) with full sentences, and even correct grammar, to get the ball rolling. If you're shy, starting out with something like "I'm excited for tonight! What are we going to do?" might be a smooth way to ease into the conversation. Little more brazen? "Tell me what you're going to do to me" might get the conversation going. No holds barred? "Tonight, I want you to eat me out until I can't take it anymore" is sure to capture pretty much anyone's attention.

Now, these are conversation openers about an upcoming date or sexual encounter. You can also send "sexts" that play out a sexual experience. Example:

You: I drop my clothes to the floor.

Them: My hands grab your breasts.

Them: Your nipples are hard, I pinch them.

*You: *gasp* God, that feels good. Kiss me.*

Them: I already am.

You: Slipping your shirt over your head.

You: Undoing your pants.

Them: How come you still have your skirt and panties on?

Them: Take them off!

You: Done. Pushing you onto the floor, so your head is near my pussy.

Them: I want to lick you so bad.

You: Not yet.

And so on and so forth. This can go on for a few minutes, or an entire day, or even a week. Some people just text, IM, or e-mail back and forth like this, while others might act out some of the actions on themselves while masturbating (taking their clothes off, pinching their nipples as their partner texted them they'd like to do).

You can even use these types of conversations as ways to negotiate what type of sexual activities you might be craving, those you want to try but have yet to bring up, or even things that you don't want to have happen. Examples:

You: Holy shit, I can't stop thinking about fucking you in the ass tonight. Tell me how hard you are!

Or

You: What would you do if I told you I wanted to tie you to the bed, blindfold you, and fuck your brains out?

Or

You: I don't want to even take my clothes off tonight, or have you touch me. I just want to worship your naked body till the sun comes up.

These are all ways to impart information about your sexual preferences to another person. Of course, if you want to use U for you and 2 for two, go for it—it can get tough to text or type with just one hand. Conversely, sometimes those texts can be hard to read, and you definitely want to make sure that your point gets across. Make the decision based on how you usually text and type, and how their text messages, e-mails, and IMs look. You can be as short and sweet or long and descriptive as you'd like.

There's No Trick to It

Some people tell me that they don't think they could ever be good at dirty talking or texting. There's no magical science to it; just say what you're thinking and feeling. You don't need it to sound like a flowery romance novel or raunchy porn to get their juices flowing. If you ever feel that you've hit a wall, just describe what's going on. "I'm so wet thinking of you." "I can't get your body out of my mind." "I wish you could take me across my office desk RIGHT NOW." See? Nothing fancy, just putting your thoughts to the keyboard.

Practice Safe Sext

With all these awesome technologies also comes some responsibility. Don't be stupid. If you know your employer monitors your keystrokes, or computers in general, don't use your work computer to send sexually related e-mails. Remember that everything is stored somewhere forever, so send your messages directly to the person you want to have see the text (or the picture)—that is, doing it through Facebook or Twitter or other social media might come back to bite you in the ass. Remember a certain congressman whose last name is slang for a penis? Make sure you have the right number or e-mail address, and that it isn't a shared family account (you probably don't want your child/roommate/business partner opening up a blow-by-blow account of what you plan to be doing to your stud muffin later that evening). If you work in a high-profile job, you might not want to send pictures with your face—again, electronics keep copies of everything. If you're doing things that might hurt you if they became public (having multiple partners, having affairs, doing kinky things that your boss/constituents might frown upon), don't document it. It seems like that should be common sense, but given what comes out in the media, that doesn't seem to be the case.

All in all, texting, sexting, IMing, and sending dirty e-mails can be fun and a huge turn-on for all parties involved. It's particularly great for some ongoing sensual foreplay leading up to a night out or for a couple who may have a long-distance relationship and need a way to keep things sizzling from opposite coasts. Just remember, an errant sexual text or photo sent to the wrong person, or a sexy and descriptive e-mail left open on a work computer, might cause repercussions, so please make sure that you think things through before hopping onto the oh-so-popular sexting bandwagon. Use it for good, not for evil (even if you had a really bad breakup), and delete things that are no longer relevant, and you should be good to go.

Super-Sensation Play!

Sensation play clearly doesn't just stop with the brain; there's a lot more to it than that. You can use all sorts of sensation on human skin to bring forth reactions of various levels of intensity. Consider removing the sense of sight (with a blindfold, scarf, etc.) to intensify the sensations that your partner is feeling even more.

When thinking about sensations on your skin, which of the following sounds the most appealing?

➤ *Soft and Fuzzy, page 91*

➤ *Hot and Cold, page 94*

➤ *Sharp and Scratchy, page 96*

➤ Soft and Fuzzy

Think back on some of your favorite memories: cuddling with a stuffed animal, curling up on the couch with a super-soft blanket, discovering those ridiculously comfortable slipper socks that feel as if they were made of Muppet fur. Our bodies, for the most part, respond well to the fluffy touch and sensation of soft and fuzzy things. It just feels that good to us. In fact, many "sex kits" come with things like satin wrist ties and feathers for tickling. This type of sensation is liked pretty much universally (although, of course, there are exceptions to any rule), so lots of people are already thinking about props they can use.

Feather Fun Forever

Feathers, of course, are some of the easiest and most sensual-looking "soft things" that one can find. While we tend to associate them with tickling (which is kind of odd, since how much legitimate tickling can you actually accomplish with a feather?), they're also wonderful for imparting light, sensual sensation onto ourselves and our partners. Have your partner lie back, naked, and gently move the feather all over their body. You can use the tip for more direct sensation and the long edge for more distributed sensation (of course, you can also use the quill for something a little more sharp and scratchy, but that's a different section in this chapter). You can use feathers from the craft store, buy ones specifically designed for sexual play, or even just use feathers and feathers on sticks from the pet store (a great game to play is Sex Toy or Cat Toy—just remember that your feline friends probably are not aware of the difference).

Please don't use feathers you've randomly picked up outside, unless you know how to clean them well. Also, make sure that whoever you're using the feather(s) on is not allergic to them. The prick of an EpiPen when you're going for something softer usually puts a crimp in your sex life.

Soft as Silk

Other things that are soft and silky can be used as well. If you have silky or satin ties, you can run them over your partner's body, use them as soft blindfolds or tie a partner up gently. (Note: Be careful though. Some knots can become super tight when you pull on them. Use scarves that you won't be sad to cut off in worst-case scenario situations. If the person being restrained is a known puller, it might be worth investing in a nice set of wrist or ankle restraints.) You can slide the scarves through their legs, and if you have one that's either washable or you're willing to part with, you can use it as part of a hand job or manual stimulation to provide a whole new sensation to the genital region.

Soft on the Wallet

The dollar store can be a great place to find fun sensation-play objects to experiment with. Gloves and cloths used to wash and wax cars are often super soft and feel amazing on the skin. Leather (and faux leather) driving gloves can offer either a fuzzier suede sensation or a smooth and cool leather sensation to the skin. Just keep in mind that because most of these cloths and materials cannot be sterilized, they should be used with only one person's genitals. This is why the dollar store is so useful—you're not spending a fortune on something that can be used for sex only with a specific person.

Fur: Faux or for Real?

They make gloves out of bunny fur that you can run over the skin, which feels amazing. If you don't want to drop that kind of cash, or are concerned about the welfare of said bunnies, you can go to the local fabric store and buy a length of fake fur. While there, you can also purchase some silk or satin fabric for the same purpose. Satin elbow-length gloves can also feel great as you slide your hands along your partner's body, and you can even use them for manual stimulation and hand jobs as you play with their genitalia.

Full Soft Circle

Just make sure that if you're going this route of soft and fuzzy toys that you continue to bring it back to sensual touch, rather than just being cozy. Encasing your partner in a super-soft blanket with fuzzy slippers might feel incredibly comfortable to them, but it also might make them sleepy, killing the mood for sexy time right then and there. It's not too tough to find a good balance, and before you know it, you might be picking out some fun, soft, and sensual items when you're out and about, giggling to yourselves about how you plan to use them.

➤ *Hot and Cold*

Long before the advent of Katy Perry's hit of the same name, people were using hot and cold sensations in the bedroom to get some sumptuous sensations going. Temperature play is not for everyone, but don't knock it until you've tried it. Some people just like cooler and cold temperatures, others just like to play with warm and hot things, while still more folks like both, even going from one extreme to the other. It depends on each person and what sensations that person's body likes to experience.

A Word of Warning

While I'm using the terms *hot* and *cold*, this doesn't mean that you should boil things or stick them in the microwave to heat them up, nor does it mean that you should put things in the freezer and then directly on someone's skin. Doing either of these could result in burns and frostbite, which doesn't make for a good time. In fact, it could make for a trip to the doctor or ER. Make sure to use some basic common sense and test the temperature of anything before you put it on someone's skin.

The Safe Way to Heat and Cool

With sex toys made of temperature-conducting materials (stainless steel, aluminum, glass, or ceramic), you definitely shouldn't be boiling them or freezing them. Instead, to warm them up, you can put them in a bowl of warm (not hot) water, let them sit for a minute or two, and then use them. If you want to cool them down, place them in a bowl of ice water for a minute or two, and then they'll be cold enough for use.

Ice, Ice Baby

Sex toys are not the only things you can use for fun temperature play. Something as easy and simple as an ice cube works well.

Make sure you let it melt a little first (or run some water on it to melt it) so that it doesn't stick to delicate skin. You can rub it all over anyone's body—from large expanses of skin to the nipples, the lips, and the genitals. Try not to leave it in any one place for too long before moving it.

You can pass it back and forth in a kiss, or suck on it to cool down your mouth before you go down on your partner. You can also make long ice cubes (look for the molds marketed to make long ice that goes into water bottles), and after they've melted a little, you can use them to penetrate yourself or your partner. If they break off inside, it's not an issue, since they'll just melt. In fact, they even make a toy called the Ice Vibe, where you freeze a vibrator into a rounded ice cube, so you end up with a vibrating ice cube to have fun with.

Getting Hot in Here

Warm and hot sensations can be fabulous, too. In addition to warming up sex toys, consider making a cup of tea and sipping some before you go down on your partner. The warm tea will heat up your mouth, and if you choose a peppermint tea, you can give some added tingles along with your hot mouth action. Another option is to either warm up massage oil before you massage it into your partner or, better yet, get yourself a massage candle. These sensual candles are made with scented soy wax, which burns at a super-low temperature. You can start burning it beforehand or at the beginning of foreplay, and it'll melt into a wonderfully warm and fabulously scented massage oil that you can then pour out onto your partner. The melted "wax" is now just soy massage oil and will absorb into the skin like any other massage oil.

Ambient Temperature Ambivalent

Something to keep in mind with temperature play is the overall temperature of wherever you're playing, and also the temperature outside. For example, you both might love cool and cold play, but using ice cubes all over the body when it's snowing outside and you're already shivering before you start might be just plain bone chilling. If you're in the dog days of summer and the thermometer is reading triple digits, pouring warm massage oil on someone might feel more like temperature torture than a sensual activity. On the other hand, if you play with heat when you're both shivering with cold or use ice cubes to cool each other down when you could fry an egg on the sidewalk, it might wind up feeling even more awesome than you thought that it would. Just remember, it's all about the communication and making sure that you're both on the same page.

Pay Attention to Piercings

If your partner has piercings, keep in mind that the metal will heat up or cool down significantly more quickly than the surrounding skin. Make sure you feel it so that it doesn't wind up getting uncomfortably hot or cold. If it does become too much, you can always use your mouth to warm that area back up again, or use an ice cube to cool it down again. Have fun, be creative, and enjoy the fabulous fun of playing with temperatures.

❧ *Sharp and Scratchy*

Oftentimes, people think of sensation play as all kinds of lovey-dovey and woo-woo, and never seem to realize that sharp can be a sensation, too. Now, we're not talking about intense knife play or drawing blood, but lots of people love the feeling of fingernails scratching down their back. If that's a sensation that you like, there are lots of similar things that you can use to help re-create that sensation, or make sensations that are similar, but go just beyond the use of fingernails.

At the Tip of Your Fingers

Fingernail scratches by themselves are great. You can drag all the nails on one hand down someone's back, or butt, or thighs (pretty much anywhere that you like or they like). You can use just one nail and delicately run it across their skin. You can carve your name into them, or let them give you goose bumps as they scratch you from head to toe.

The key here is to make sure that both of you have CLEAN fingernails. As a society, we don't clean under our nails as much as we should, letting them turn into a haven for dirt and bacteria. While this is usually not too much of an issue, when you scratch someone (or are scratched by them) you can transfer that dirt and bacteria, and if the scratches end up a little too deep, they can get infected from this unintentional transfer. The easy solution is to make sure that you keep your fingernails nice and clean. Lots of soap and warm water should help, and if you know that you're a deep scratcher (or that your partner is), it may be worth it to get a fingernail brush.

What Else?

Lots of sharp and pokey things can be co-opted into your sex life. Bamboo skewers or toothpicks both make fabulously fun scratching toys that are then easily discarded. They're particularly good if you have multiple partners, because you don't have to worry about cleaning them. They're also great for travel, because they're safe for airplanes and disposable. If sharing and traveling are not on your list of things to worry about, buying a nice metal skewer to use for scratching in the bedroom can be great—just make sure to designate it a sex toy or clean it well if you plan to use it in the kitchen and the bedroom.

Like fingernails, and even knives for that matter, skewers and toothpicks can be used either very lightly and gently to just barely scratch the skin's surface or with significantly more pressure to create deeper marks, or even to break the skin. As with everything, make sure that you both communicate your wants, needs, and expectations around using these toys, and always start lighter—it's much easier to increase pressure but much more difficult to "take back" something you've already done.

Living on the Edge

This brings us to knives. Now, I'm not suggesting that you bring a giant butcher knife into the bedroom (unless, of course, that's what you want to do, and in that case, I just urge that you take safety measures into consideration). In fact, you can get adorably cute little hunting and carving knives. You can use them to GENTLY run down the skin without even making a mark, or press down with a more even pressure to use the tip for scratching. You can also flip knives over and use the backside—it creates many of the same sensations that people tend to enjoy, but without the risk of accidentally cutting someone, so it's a safer choice, especially for folks new to the knife world.

A great trick if you're a little nervous about *actually* using a knife on someone is to show them the knife, and then blindfold them. Once they're blindfolded, take a pen that's out of ink or the edge of a credit card and run that down their skin. Although these edges are not nearly as sharp as a knife, they feel similar enough, especially when the mind has already seen and processed the idea that a knife is going to be used. The same reaction (shivers, goose bumps, excitement, etc.) comes across, and no one is the wiser to the fact that you never used the knife.

Better Than a Winning Scratch Off

Lastly, there are more scratchy sensations. Think of the feel of rough calluses across your skin, or even something a bit more abrasive like sandpaper. Some people love this feeling, and some hate it. Try it out and see what you and your partner like. A trip to the dollar store can come up with rough cloths, scrubby brushes, steel wool, and other objects to create that sensation on different levels of intensity.

Chapter

7

Toys for Big Girls and Boys – Sex Toys and Lube

Sex toys and personal lubricants: They're not just the stuff of creepy adult stores and seedy arcades on the edge of town. Various studies have shown that anywhere from 50 to 75 percent of American women like using a sex toy either on their own or with a partner, so it's time to get with the program and pick up some lube and sex toys of your own.

I can't say it enough; it's perfectly normal and natural for people to use lubricant and sex toys, whether they're getting themselves off or having sex with a partner. Needing lube or a little extra love from a toy doesn't mean that there's anything wrong with the person wanting it, it doesn't mean that you're not attracted to your partner, and it doesn't mean that either of you is doing anything wrong. What it DOES mean is that everyone involved in the sexual adventuring has a vested interested in making sure that everyone has a rocking good time, whatever it may take to get there. So now, as I step off this sex toy–loving soapbox, I invite you to learn as much as you like about the truly delightful world of sex toys and lubricants, and figure out exactly what it is that might kick your motor into high gear.

This chapter covers three different areas:

X--- Talking about toys: Are you a newbie, almost ready to rock, or a stockholder in sex toys?

X--- Couples' toys: Do you like the sound of a vibrator, a dildo, or something more unique?

X--- Learning to love lube: Which lube is right for you? Water-based, silicone-based, or oil-based?

Talking about Toys

When you begin to consider bringing sex toys into the bedroom, which of the following is closest to how you might identify yourself?

> ❥ *A Toyland Newbie, page 102*

> ❥ *I'm Almost Ready to Rock, page 105*

> ❥ *A Stockholder in Sex Toys, page 107*

❥ *A Toyland Newbie*

You hear the term "sex toy" and are either completely befuddled or the only image that enters your brain is that of Charlotte's addiction to her Rabbit vibrator on *Sex and the City*. The idea of beginning a sex toy collection might seem a bit overwhelming to start with, but once you learn more about toys and how you can use them, either on your own or with a partner, you'll be an expert in no time.

Not Everyone Has the Same Vibe

Probably the most frequently discussed sex toy is the vibrator (yes, Charlotte DID have one). While Charlotte made the Rabbit-style vibrator so famous, it turns out that the Rabbit-style toy (not all are rabbits; there are dolphins, and butterflies, and panthers, and I've even seen those with beavers and cobras, as well as less animal-focused options) doesn't work well for all women's bodies. In fact, a good number of women have desperately tried to find the right Rabbit-style toy that stimulates them internally while also being perfectly positioned to give their clit some awesome loving, and have felt that the failure was theirs when these toys didn't do their duty. This is a case of "it's not you, it's them."

Rabbit-style vibes tend to be made in a one-sex-fits-all category that many find overwhelming. Instead, check out the many clitoral vibes — the Pocket Rocket, the LELO Mia, the LELO Siri (no connection to the iPhone), the Je Joue Mimi, the Waterdancer, or the Fun Factory Layaspot — to find one that you like the look of, like the options on, and can be positioned wherever you'd like. You can also check out internal vibrators — like the Je Joue G-Ki, the LELO Gigi, the Fun Factory Elle, the LELO Liv — or even combine an external and an internal vibe to create your own dual-vibration stimulation that fits you and your body the way that you want them to.

Pass on the Jelly

Any vibrator (or other sex toy) made from a jelly material (also called sil-a-gel, gelee, Jel-ee, etc.) is not safe for use on your body. This material contains something called phthalates, which are rubber softeners (like what they use on shower curtains), and not only do they smell bad, but they can leach into your body during use, causing irritation, pain, and even potentially, cancer. Stick with sex toy materials that are phthalate-free, like hard plastic, elastomer, TPR, medical grade silicone, glass, metal, ceramic, corian, stone, and wood. If something smells bad and you wouldn't want to put it in your mouth, you probably shouldn't be putting it anywhere else either.

The Big (or Little) D

In addition to vibrators, we have dildos, which, while they can vibrate, are more designed for internal use, and many of which are also compatible with harnesses, so that you can strap it on and penetrate your partner or so that they can strap it on and penetrate you. People of all genders and orientations can use harnesses and dildos, and they can be used vaginally or anally (or even for oral sex). If you don't have a partner at hand, a dildo can be manually used by yourself for penetration, or can be held and used by a partner as part of sexual activity. Friendly dildo companies include Vixen Creations, Tantus, Happy Valley, Fun Factory, Whipspider Rubberworks, and others that make 100 percent medical grade silicone dildos.

Backdoor Presents

There are lots of different anal sex toys, which are discussed in-depth in the anal chapter, including anal dildos, butt plugs, anal beads, anal probes, and more. Anything used in the anus should have a flared base (wider than the rest of the toy) to keep it from slipping inside your body and getting stuck. Also, toys used anally should be designated for your butt, used with a condom, or made of a sterilizable material. Even in the same body, anal bacteria can cause oral and vaginal infections, so make sure that you keep things clean.

Paging Dr. Kegel

Another group of "sex toys," which are really more "sexual health toys," are those that help strengthen your vaginal muscles (often called PC muscles or Kegel muscles). Having strong pelvic floor muscles can lead to longer, stronger, and more intense orgasms, less issues with bladder control (including during pregnancy and aging), easier recovery after vaginal birth, and other benefits. Basically, having strong Kegel muscles makes you that much more awesome! While you can do Kegel exercises on your own, you can also get Kegel balls that, once inserted, help your body to do these exercises subconsciously when you're moving. These are NOT Ben Wa Balls (small metal balls meant to be worn during intercourse and moved around with your Kegel muscles), but balls specifically designed to be worn for hours at a time, allowing you to build stronger Kegel muscles.

Some of the great options out there include Fun Factory Smart Balls (available with one ball or two, depending on your vagina size and whether you may have a tilted uterus), the Je Joue Ami (which has three sets in different sizes/weights, so you can work your way up as you get stronger and stronger), and the LELO

Luna beads (which also have two weight options). So work out in a way that will literally improve your sex life, and everyone involved will be happy!

Knowledge Is Power

Of course, there are more sex toys—from kinkier items (discussed in chapter 11) to items that make you scratch your head (look up "The Magic Banana" online; no, I can't figure it out either)—but this is a basic 101 for you. Now you can feel comfortable going into a brightly lit sex toy store, or if you're not ready for that, you can browse some sex toy websites. Heck, even Amazon.com and Walgreens.com sell sex toys now, although I'd suggest that you buy from an actual sex toy store, which will have better information and selection. Go forth and use sex toys to your best advantage!

❥ *I'm Almost Ready to Rock*

So you've discovered sex toys. Maybe you've glimpsed the positive change that they can bring to your love life (or your single life). While maybe you have a vibrator or two, or even a butt plug, perhaps you're not sure what else you might need to add to your collection to truly be a sex toy rock star. Or maybe you want more information on sex toy materials, storage, and so on. Don't worry; we have you covered.

Your Toy Box

Shall we talk a bit about sex toy storage? I mean, if you have only a vibe or two, it doesn't matter that much where you keep them. In all likelihood, you just throw it in the drawer of a nightstand or tuck it in among your underthings. Once you begin a bona fide sex toy collection, it's time to rethink how you want to store and even organize your toys, both so that they're kept in good condition and so that you can find what you want when you want it.

Here are some things to keep in mind: don't store glass toys (or ceramic or metal toys) where they can knock into each other. This is one way to chip your favorite toy, and bench it for life. (Note: This SHOULD go without saying, but if you break or chip a glass toy, please don't try to fix it. It's no longer viable as a toy and shouldn't be used on or in your genitals. Ever. Please and thank you.) Most glass toys come in a fancy bag from the maker, or at least something to keep them from getting chipped or broken en route. Keep that, or you can make your own bags, but don't just throw all your glass toys into a pile together. You'll absolutely regret it later.

Ditto goes for storing silicone (or any soft toys) together, even though the issue here is less about chipping than about melting and creating one massive Godzilla zombie sex toy. You may think that I'm joking, but storing silicone toys together is a bad idea. The different types of silicone all want to be the same, and so they actually change their makeup, ending up with a melted cheese–like texture, and melting into the other toys. Consider purchasing a little plastic bin for each toy. You can also wrap them in fabric (bandanas work well), or make them each little cloth baggies. If you have enough toys to warrant it (and don't mind giving up one side of your closet or bedroom door), an over-the-door shoe holder is perfect for storing a vibrator, dildo, or anal toy in each little pouch. Don't store your sex toys in plastic baggies even if the toys are clean going in. Any bacteria that might get trapped in there when you seal it can multiply and either ruin your toy or just be plain gross.

Sharing Your Toys

Planning on using your toy(s) with multiple partners? Make sure you buy materials that can be sterilized, or use a condom every time you use the toy. Sterilizable materials include 100 percent medical grade silicone (if it smells, it is NOT silicone), glass, metal, and ceramic. To clean a toy for personal use, or for use with a monogamous partner, soap and warm water work well. You don't need to buy fancy toy cleaner; soap and water are good enough for general cleaning regularly.

To sterilize a toy (to deep clean it for use with a new partner or to prevent yourself from recontracting your own urinary tract infection or yeast infection, which can happen), you'll want to boil it for three to five minutes, run it through the dishwasher on the top shelf, or wipe it down with a 10 percent bleach solution (10 percent bleach, 90 percent water), let it dry, and then wash it off again with soap and water. Don't use alcohol on silicone or soft toys: it can dry them out or damage them.

Get Creative

There are no real rules about sex toys (except that if it's going in your butt, it needs to have a flanged base), so feel free to get creative and experiment. It's fine to use a clitoral/external vibrator on your nipples, or an internal vibrator on your clitoris. Heck, the Hitachi Magic Wand (the Cadillac of vibrators) is sometimes sold as a neck massager. So do what you want with all your sex toys, and figure out what works best for you. No rules, just awesome sexy time. Have fun!

✦ *A Stockholder in Sex Toys*

You know what's up. You've moved beyond the vibrator basics, and there are no Rabbits or Pocket Rockets in your collection.

Perhaps you can list your favorite brands by name (LELO, Tantus, Vixen, Je Joue, Fun Factory ... the list goes on!), and maybe you've even written a sex toy review or two yourself. You know that there are three types of power for vibrators: rechargeable (either USB or AC/DC), batteries, and plug-in (a.k.a. weapons grade sex toys, like everyone's favorite, the Hitachi Magic Wand). You know how to clean your sex toy (mild soap and water for regular use, and either boiling, the dishwasher, or a 10 percent bleach solution for a deep clean). You have a sex toy storage system so that they're easy to find and not touching ... so why are you reading this section?

Do Your Toys Pass the Test?

Maybe you want to know more about materials, and whether companies are telling the truth about what they're putting on the market. A new nonprofit called Dildology had the same thought: it was created solely to act as an independent testing agency to corroborate (or call out) companies that say they're making body-friendly sex toys out of body-friendly material. Donors can suggest toys for testing, and they'll support the testing and release the results. Their site is definitely worth checking out at dildology.com.

You might also enjoy learning more from the Coalition Against Toxic Toys, a group working to educate people all over the world about sex toys and sex toy materials, and how there's no regulation of them. They also list educators and sex toy stores that offer body-friendly, nontoxic sex toys, and sometimes share info about sex toy buyback and recycling programs for those toys you bought and now won't put in your body because they smell like death (or because you happen to know that they're chock-full o' phthalates).

Spread the Good Word!

Otherwise, go forth into the world, sex toy goddess! Share your knowledge with your friends and family, let people know the positive difference that good-quality sex toys can make in someone's sex life, and how it can completely change how someone might feel about sex. Make sure that people know to stay away from toys that contain evil phthalates, and make sure that they know how to clean and store their toys for expanding their toys' lives. It's up to you to spread the joy that is the wonderful world of sex toys!

Couples' Toys

All right, so we've got the basics of sex toys, what they are, and how they work. Now let's talk about getting them into bed with your partner.

Lots of people think sex toys are for use only while you're flying solo, clicking the five-finger mouse, ringing southern bells, and so on (I'm talking about masturbation, in case you're wondering). To that, I say pish posh. Did you know that only 33 percent of heterosexual women can climax during intercourse alone? Same thing goes for all women during JUST penetration with no other stimulation of any kind. Not adding in some sex toys to the equation can leave you feeling a bit lacking in the orgasm department. I mean, sure, oral sex can solve some of those problems, but adding a vibrator can make things better for everyone … and of course, the vibrator is not the only sex toy option that can be added to couples' time to turn up the heat!

If you're worried about introducing sex toys to your partner, I suggest that you go sex toy shopping together. Of course, it could be fun to introduce a new addition as a surprise one evening in bed, but that may be a trigger for some people and may make them feel that you think that they're inadequate. To deal with this, try going to the toy store together and pick out something that feels perfect to you both, or take some time to sit down together to do your online shopping, so that you can both feel invested in the toy(s) that you've picked out, and neither of you will feel that something was sprung on you without your consent. Now, if you've already talked about it (or already used sex toys together), there's a lot more wiggle room about picking out a fun new item to let your lover know that you were thinking of them.

So how do you choose the right toy for you and yours? Would you say that you prefer:

- ❥ *The Buzz of a Vibe, page 110*
- ❥ *The Feel of a Dildo, page 112*
- ❥ *Something More Unique, page 119*

❥ *The Buzz of a Vibe*

Millions of couples around the world use vibrators as part of their sex time. There's nothing wrong with adding a vibrator to your time together, and it can optimize your sexual interactions, and in some cases save your love life. Think about it. If you both enjoy intercourse (regardless of the genders of those involved), but at least one of you cannot climax from it (like two-thirds of women), how often are you going to want to keep having intercourse? However, if you get a vibrator that can make it so that everyone involved is feeling all types of pleasure (and potentially so that everyone involved is able to orgasm if they so desire), then think about how that changes the conversation about sex.

Vibes for the Outside

Clitoral vibes (sometimes referred to as an external vibrator) are great couples' toys because they have so many ways that they can be used. Of course, using it to stimulate the clitoris and labia is a great option, but you can also use it on other parts, to stimulate nipples, the pubic bone of either party, even up and down on the scrotum. Regardless of the type of sex toy, either you or your partner can hold it in place. Many are designed to be positioned between bodies during intercourse, but they could also be used during oral sex. You could use it before sex, during sex, or after sex. You could masturbate next to each other in bed, or use the vibrator to manually stimulate each other if you're up to some handiwork. Again, no rules around sex toys if they're not going in your butt, so get creative and figure out what works best for both you and your partner!

Is Using a Vibrator Still "Real" Sex?

One of the most frequently voiced concerns around vibrators, especially those being used in a longtime relationship, is whether someone can get addicted to a vibrator and never be able to have "real" sex again. Note that "real" is in quotation marks—lots of people's REAL sex lives involve the use of various sex toys, often including vibrators. The fear is that someone will either get desensitized because of a vibrator and will no longer enjoy the sensation that their partner's hands/mouth/tongue/penis/what have you can provide, or that they'll get addicted to the vibrator's sensations and not ever want anything else. Folks, vibrators don't kiss, cuddle, or spoon. They don't take you on dates or take out the trash. While there certainly are jokes about B.O.B. (the battery-operated boyfriend), no one wants to end up in a long-term relationship (or even a friendly with-benefits situation) with a vibrator. Period.

That said, many women cannot orgasm without help from their vibrator. Oral sex might feel great, but they need something more vibrational to climax. This doesn't mean that they don't enjoy sex with their partners—it just means that they need a little extra help to get over the edge. If someone does feel that they're getting desensitized because of their vibrator use, they can stop using it for a few days, weeks, or months, and eventually their body will return to the sensitivity level it was at. There's no reason to be scared of someone leaving their lover to elope with a vibrator. It simply doesn't happen (and if it ever did, my guess would be that there were a lot of other issues in that relationship aside from just the vibrator).

❥ *The Feel of a Dildo*

You're in it deep, and are hungry for depth. Sounds like a dildo is right up your alley. Dildos are made of all sorts of materials: jelly (stay away or always use a condom on this type of material), silicone, glass, aluminum, steel, marble, granite, corian, ceramics, and even wood. (No, it's not like putting a tree branch inside you—think more like a salad bowl. Wooden dildos are sanded down and covered with a polyurethane coating to make them safe for use inside bodies.) Before you decide what type of dildo the two of you might want, you need to figure out what you want to do with it.

Getting Strapped On

If either one of you (or even both of you!) is going to be strapping it on with a harness, you're going to want a silicone dildo, period.

Hard materials are not designed for use in harnesses, and you can cause damage that way because the person wearing the harness has a lot less control over their speed and depth and less ability to feel their partner's reaction than they would with a penis. If someone's going to be strapping it on, you'll want not only a silicone dildo but one with a base that lets it fit and stay snug within a harness. Coincidentally, dildos that are harness compatible are also automatically OK for anal use, because of their flanged base. Keep in mind that anyone can be penetrated anally, and anyone can wear a harness to penetrate their partner, regardless of their genitals and orientation.

Let's talk a little bit about picking out a harness and a dildo that together create the fabulous combo that we frequently refer to as "a strap-on" — although really, there is no such sex toy as "a strap-on" by itself.

Harness Materials

You can find harnesses in a huge variety of sizes, styles, and materials. Of course, there's no one perfect harness that's right for everyone across the board, but there's probably one that happens to be just right for you. Harness materials can include leather, pleather, vinyl, nylon webbing with faux velvet, just nylon webbing, swimsuit-like material, rope, rubber, and even a few additional options (a small company in Seattle makes harnesses out of recycled bike tires!).

Make sure you think about material when choosing your harness. If you're a vegan, you'll want to stay away from the leather. If it's important to you to be able to drop it in the washing machine, you'll want something made of swimsuit material or nylon webbing. Got more than one partner and will be sharing? Clearly, you'll want a harness that can be sterilized, like vinyl, not leather.

Want something that looks a little more kinky or fetish? Leather or rubber might be the perfect solution. Some people have multiple harnesses of different materials, either for different partners or different activities.

Note: Different harnesses (styles, brands, etc.) fit different sizes. If you're curvier, make sure it adjusts to fit your hips. If you're slimmer, make sure you can get it tight enough. If you and your partner are planning on purchasing one harness and taking turns, look for a harness that's adjustable to both of your body sizes.

Harness Styles

The two most common styles are the thong (a.k.a. the single-strap or G-string harness) and the jock. The thong style goes around your hips and has just one strap that runs between your legs. This style is much better for those with vulvas than those with penises—it kind of presses the penis and testicles in half and is never comfortable. A lot of women enjoy the thong style because it offers some clitoral rubbing while you're wearing it. Conversely, a fair number of folks don't like this style because they either don't like the feeling of a thong or want more access to their own vulva so that their partner can play with it during sex. Some of the more popular thong-style harnesses are Sportsheets Bare as You Dare, SpareParts Theo, and some of the Jaguars by ASLAN Leather.

The jock style (a.k.a. the two-strap) harness has two leg straps that fit firmly around your butt cheeks; it kind of looks like you're wearing a stylized jock strap. Pros and cons aside, everyone's ass looks AMAZING in this type of harness. Period. Some harness users might feel that this style is too sporty for them, but others love the support it provides, the ability to have multiple straps to adjust, and of course, the access it provides to the wearer's genitals during sex. Popular versions of the two-strap harness include SpareParts Joque, SpareParts Corsette Vibrating Harness, Outlaw's Annie-O, Stormy Leather's Terra Firma, and Stockroom's La Femme.

Now, those are the two easiest-to-find harness styles, but they certainly aren't the only options. In fact, there's a plethora of other harness choices out there, should you wish to experiment. Some companies make palm harnesses for those well versed in handiwork (hey, your hand CAN get tired after a while), and others offer a thigh harness, perfect for sex while spooning or if you want to pin your lover up against the wall and penetrate them easily while standing (also great for people with mobility issues!). There's also a whole list of chest harnesses, boot harnesses, chin harnesses, forehead harnesses, and more; you can strap it on in as many ways as you can possibly imagine!

Talking about Dildos

Next, we have the other half of the whole strap-on combo: the sex toy that actually fits in the harness, allowing you to stand proud and tall, and even penetrate your partner with it, if you so wish. Officially (as official as you can get with sex toys), this is called a dildo, but people have come up with a ridiculous number of awesome synonyms. If you don't feel that dildo is fitting, try out cock, dong, woo-woo, Mr. Happy, Penis #2, or faux penis. Like every other type of sexual terminology, there's not one word that's right or wrong. Just choose whichever word (or set of words) makes you and your partner hot. The end.

Names You Can Trust

We've talked about the best sex toy materials throughout the book, and some companies that have expressed dedication to making phthalate-free, completely silicone toys are Tantus, Happy Valley, Vixen Creations, Whipspider Rubberworks, Vamp Silicone, and Fun Factory. If you buy their dildos, you can rest assured that they're body safe and sterilizable, in case you want to use them with multiple partners.

Which Dildo Will Do?

As with pretty much every type of sex toy, dildos are available in many sizes, shapes, colors, and designs. It's the flat base (and silicone material, as discussed above) that will allow you to use it in your harness; as long as it has that flared base, you can choose whichever dildo your heart (or other body part) desires. When picking out a dildo, make sure you talk with the person being penetrated. One of you might have a fantasy of your strap-on cock being twelve inches and flesh toned, while the other partner is dreaming of something much more petite and featuring silver sparkles. In general, our eyes tend to be bigger than our genitals. And it's always easier to go back and get something with more size; it's MUCH more difficult to make your brand-new dildo a bit smaller. Think ahead about this.

Aside from size, you need to think about whether the two of you want something realistic or a bit more fantastical. Some folks think a dildo that looks like a unicorn horn (yes, they make them) is a dream come true, while others are craving a dildo much more true to life—a caramel color with lifelike veins and balls. Like everything, there's no perfect dildo for everyone, but ensuring that both of you are on the same page about size and appearance will make everyone more satisfied in the end (literally).

Shape and texture can be important as well. Some dildos are curved for G-spot or prostate stimulation, but that might not feel awesome for some uses. As always, make sure to communicate and find a compromise that gets you both going. There are dildos that come with a vibrating bullet in the base that can be removed if desired. That being said, if the toy that's perfect for you happens to NOT have a vibrating bullet, you can always buy one separately and tuck it into your harness, or add a vibrating cock ring, if having vibration is important to you.

The Double D

One last type of dildo to consider is the updated double-ended dildo. The original ones that looked like jelly javelins were useless to most women; unless you're super bendy (or possibly ridiculously creative), the best you can do with one is to use it as a javelin in your local sex Olympics. However, things have changed. Some of the companies creating sex toys realized the futility of using a long stick for two bodies and have now created the oh-so-popular modern double-ended dildos.

They come in two options: the first is two differently sized and differently shaped dildos stuck together in a V shape, and the second looks like a longer dildo with a large bulb on the end. Both are used the same way. The user places one end (from the V-shaped style) or the bulb in their vagina or anus, and using their muscles to hold it in place, places the other end in their partner's vagina or anus (using lube, obviously), and then goes for the gold. Men can choose to wear these if they have erectile dysfunction, or they can use them along with their penis to provide their partner with double penetration, if said partner has both a vulva and an anus. Basically, anyone can wear them to penetrate any gender of partner that they may have. Oddly enough, some folks call these toys "strapless strap-ons," although many people wind up using them along with their harnesses to keep them steady and prevent the end worn inside the penetrator from popping out during sex.

Some of the more popular double dildos available on the market are the Feeldoe by Tantus, the Nexus by Vixen Creations, the Sysil by Mantric, and the Share by Fun Factory, most of which come in different sizes, shapes, and colors, like single dildos, to make sure that you and your partner are satisfied in every possible way.

Sans Strap-on
If you're not going to be using the dildo in a harness, but rather to penetrate each other, or even to penetrate yourself in front of your partner, then you have unlimited options of material and can use any of those listed above. Materials like glass, metal, stone, and ceramic are great for temperature play if you or your partner like having things nice and warm or cool and chilly. Please keep in mind that you should never boil, freeze, or microwave a dildo before using it on someone (including yourself!); third-degree burns or frostbite put a quick end to any sexual adventure. Instead, you can warm up or cool down sex toys by placing them in a bowl of warm water or ice water, changing the temperature without creating a dangerous environment for anyone's nether regions.

An Addition to Oral
Some people like to be penetrated during oral sex, and with cunnilingus, using a dildo can be easier to manage (and be longer and wider than fingers), so that's a great option. You can also use it to penetrate a partner anally, either during oral sex or during intercourse. If they have both a vulva and an anus, then a dildo can help make double penetration (if all parties agree) a reality without bringing in a third person, or someone with a penis might want a little anal action while they're penetrating their partner. Again, if you can think of it, there are countless ways to integrate

dildos into your love life, and all of them can be fabulous and fun for you and your partner or partners.

❥ *Something More Unique*

More sex toys, please! Your bedroom sex toy collection doesn't need to be limited to dildos and vibrators when there are so many other fantastic options at hand. Of course, we have all the anal and butt toy options, but they'll all be discussed in the anal section. Feel free to add in butt plugs, anal beads, and more to increase pleasure in the posterior department as you see fit.

If You Like It, Put a Ring on It

If your partner has a penis, cock rings (sometimes called penis rings or c-rings) can be your best friends. They're also available in multiple types of materials from stretchy jelly to firmer silicone, and even in metal and leather options. When starting out, go with jelly or silicone, as they're stretchier and easier to remove (jelly is OK in these toys, as they're not used inside the body). There are also leather options that snap on and off, which could be a good choice as well. They come in both vibrating and non-vibrating varieties—the ones that vibrate will give him some extra sensation, as well as you if you're being penetrated while he's wearing the vibrating ring.

So here's the big trick that everyone seems to miss out on: put the ring on when he's still at least semi-flaccid (soft or not fully erect), and put it on over BOTH the shaft of the penis AND the testicles. If you put it just on the shaft of the penis, it likely won't be tight enough and won't serve much of a purpose. If you get it on over BOTH the cock and the balls, it allows blood flow into the penis without allowing it back out again, letting it become harder for a bit longer, and when there's a climax, it's usually stronger and more intense. Especially when you're first starting out, don't have anyone wear the ring for more than twenty to twenty-five minutes. This can lead to issues with blood flow or circulation, and could end up with a trip to the emergency room. AWKWARD!

Kinkier Toys

Other toys that you can use as a couple include kink toys (nipple clamps, paddles, floggers, blindfolds, restraints, etc.), which obviously will be covered in the section on, you guessed it, kink and kinky play. Massage candles with warm wax that turns into massage oil are great couples' toys, although not often thought of as sex toys.

A Vibrating League of Its Own

There's a brilliant vibrator out there that's so unique, it clearly belongs in this section. It's called the We-Vibe. It's shaped like the letter "C" so that one end goes inside and vibrates the G-spot, and the other end stays outside and vibrates the clit. Now, while this concept is great by itself, the two things that make it truly brilliant are that first, it's made to be worn DURING PENETRATION, so that the woman can get G-spot AND clitoral vibrational stimulation during vaginal penetration or intercourse. And second, the newest model comes with a remote. Because the rechargeable vibrator holds about a two-hour charge, you could wear it out to dinner or dancing as foreplay, and hand the remote over to your partner. Ditto for during oral sex: have the person receiving oral sex hold the remote, and the person giving oral sex wear the We-Vibe. You can create a positive sex-feedback loop by having the receiver increase vibrations when whatever the giver is doing feels particularly good. Positively brilliant, no?

Learning to Love the Lube

It's time to talk about lube. There's a lot of stigma out there about personal lubricant. Some folks say that if you need to or want to use lube, it means that you're not properly turned on or that your partner isn't doing something right. All of that is total baloney. Lube helps make OK sex good and good sex great. Seriously folks, lube is love. Say it, think it, memorize it, and use it. Using lube has the ability to transform your love life.

Why Should Someone Use Lube?

Let me count the reasons. Sexual lubricant is an important part of various types of sex, and it's clear to see why. Lubrication makes all kinds of touch feel better below the belt, both outside on the lips, clitoris, and hood, all over the penis and scrotum, as well as inside the vagina or anus, whether you're using fingers, tongues, or toys. It can help reduce friction too, which makes things feel better (and reduces the risk of sexually transmitted infections and irritated genitals). Seriously — put it to the test. Do a little stroking of a vulva or penis without lube, and then add a little and feel the difference. Amazing, right?

It doesn't end there. The use of lube will help transmit all sorts of sensations more intensely, which can lower the amount of effort required of the person providing those very sensations. If you're penetrating a partner, lube makes it easier and smoother to go in and out (ditto if you're the one being penetrated). Plus, if penetration of any kind is on the menu for your sexual adventure, adding some lube will definitely help prevent or reduce soreness, plus it can work to prevent tearing of the delicate vaginal and anal tissues.

Wanting Lube Does NOT Mean That You Aren't Turned On

Since most vulvas lubricate on their own, either a little or a lot, folks might be wondering why anyone might need a little extra outside lube. This is the breakdown: the amount of lube produced by someone doesn't always directly correlate to how turned on they are — meaning that someone could be revved up and ready to go in every sense of the word, yet have little to no lubricant being produced by their body, while another person may be producing lubricant for days, but her mind is more focused on whether she paid her parking meter and isn't thinking about sex at all. Clearly, the amount of lubrication isn't even close to an accurate indication of arousal. The answer someone gives when you ask them if they're ready for you to do fabulously naughty things to them is a much better indication of whether they're ready to get it on than how much lube they're producing. If you're worried about what your partner might think about using lube, have them read a little bit of this section.

So while it's true that most vulvas have the ability to lubricate naturally, there are several things that can affect natural lubrication — this results in a less than lubricated vagina (vaginas are never completely dry; they retain moisture in their mucosal membrane at all times to help your body clean itself out regularly).

What are some of these things that can lead to a vagina not having the natural lube that it needs? Everything from hormonal birth control (the patch, the pill, the ring, the Implanon, the shot) to antihistamines (any allergy medication, both prescription and over-the-counter), and yes, even stress (which tends to affect anyone capable of breathing). Add to this the fact that sometimes sexual playtime can last for hours on end. Now, it becomes clear that there are lots of reasons someone might want to add a little lube to their playtime.

Use Lube — No Ifs, Ands, or BUTTS about It

And butts? Never ever, ever, ever go there without lubrication. Not ever. Any time you're putting anything in, near, around, or next to an anus (yours or someone else's), you absolutely need to make sure that lube is part of the picture. Without using lube for anal play, you have a high likelihood of tearing delicate anal tissue, which in addition to causing pain can increase the risk of STI transmission and can even end up giving the owner of the anus a bacterial infection. Use lube, and you won't lose out.

There are three main types of lubes. Pick the one that sounds the most fun to you!

- ❥ *Water-based Lubes, page 123*
- ❥ *Silicone-based Lubes, page 125*
- ❥ *Oil-based Lubes and Massage Oils, page 127*

❥ *Water-based Lubes*

The first lube that's friendly for internal use and most frequently found is *water-based lubricant*. When people think of drugstore-bought lube, this is probably the type they're thinking of. Water-based lube is the universal donor of lubricants; it's compatible with pretty much everything: all materials that sex toys are made of; all types of condoms, gloves, and dams; and almost everybody. You want a lube that's lye-free (and glycerin- and paraben-free doesn't hurt). Some well-known brands that fit this qualification include Sliquid, Maximus, Wet Naturals, Pink Water, and Blossom Organics.

Too Sweet

Be aware of what the ingredients in your lube are; some flavored water-based lubricants contain *sugar*. For the love of vulvas, please NEVER ever use a lubricant with sugar in it near the vulva. Doing so is pretty much asking the gods of sex for a yeast infection. Although the packaging doesn't always list the ingredients, lubes containing sugar are usually sold for novelty use only, and, while they can be a fine option for blowjobs, lubes with any sugar should definitely be kept away from the vagina and the anus.

Despite the Bush Song, Glycerin Is No Good

Yet another frequently found ingredient in water-based lubes is glycerin. Overall, glycerin is a safe ingredient used in soaps, shampoos, and many health and beauty products. The problem? Many vulvas and especially vaginas seem to have a negative reaction to glycerin. Depending on the person, it can cause itching or an allergic reaction, and some folks can experience yeast infections or irritation. If you or your partner ever has these sensations after using a water-based lubricant that contains glycerin, try out a glycerin-free option, such as those listed above.

How Much to Use

So how much lube should you use, and how often should you apply it? The answer is simple; you can use as much lube as you want. If for some reason you have too much, it's easy to wipe away, but not having enough lube can result in uncomfortable irritation, and that can mean that people want sex less because it doesn't feel good. Don't fall victim to not enough lube!

When you use a water-based lube, be aware that the water can be absorbed and may evaporate, as though it were drying out. If you're like the average person, your first inclination is to add more lube to re-up. The issue here is that is the lube will just make it stickier and stickier, until you're web slinging à la Spiderman. Rather than adding more of the lube itself, just reactivate the existing lube by adding a bit of water. There are lots of options — you can use spit, try pouring some water from a cup, glass, or bottle, jump into the shower, or even attempt a mister or squirt gun. Do whatever is fun for you and your partner — some options might even turn you both on!

Food Is Not Lube

A word of warning — upon hearing about flavored lube and how fun it is to use (which it totally is), some folks might think that other things can be used instead, like chocolate syrup, whipped cream, sweet liqueurs, and so on. Just the opposite: all these things contain sugar as a main ingredient. As I discussed above, placing sugar on, near, in, or anywhere by the vulva (and sometimes also the anus) is an open invitation for a yeast infection. Don't worry — I'm not saying that you absolutely CANNOT have someone eat an ice cream sundae from on top of your vulva, but if you want that to happen, may I suggest using a layer of plastic kitchen wrap between you and the pile o' sugar? Either that, or be prepared to visit the gynecologist and start a round of antibiotics. Of course, penises tend to be a little less touchy about these things, so if you want to turn a penis into the whipped cream Tower of Pisa, be my guest.

❧ Silicone-based Lubes

Good news; there's yet another type of lube that's perfect for use internally. This kind is a *silicone-based lubricant.* Some well-known brands include Wet Platinum, Eros Bodyglide, Pjur Bodyglide, Gun Oil (not actually oil-based, contrary to its name), and Pink. Silicone lube is friendly for the vagina, anus, and penis, but is definitely not for use with silicone toys (or to be honest, any soft or squishy sex toy). It sounds counterintuitive, but using a silicone-based lube with a silicone toy will ruin it—both types of silicone want to be the same, so the toy will get all gooey, and the lube will harden, and BAM: melted cheese–like sex toy. No fun for anyone, especially your sex toy.

OK, Good, Great!
A bonus of silicone-based lube is that it's hypoallergenic, and quality silicone lube contains only a few ingredients, so it's easy to read the list and know what you're putting into your body. While it's totally safe to ingest, it's not the most delicious of the lubricants available. It can be a fabulous lube for use with manual stimulation prior to, during, or after oral sex (or on its own!), vaginal intercourse, anal stimulation, anal intercourse, hand jobs, and so on. More good news: silicone-based lubes are 100 percent safe to use with any type of condoms, gloves, and dams.

Think Energizer Bunny
If you're using a silicone-based lube, it keeps going and going and going, so you probably won't need to reapply or reactivate (this is what makes it awesome for sex in pools, hot tubs, ponds, rivers, lakes, showers, rainstorms, etc.).

There are also all sorts of other uses you can find for silicone lubes, like using it for massages, putting it on squeaky doors, calming down frizzy hair (way cheaper than many of the expensive silicone hair products that turn out to be the exact same thing), shining latex, making tattoos really pop, and more. Oh! If you or anyone you know gets irritation between their thighs when it's hot, silicone lube is basically the same thing as runner's glide. Problem solved. Silicone lube: it isn't just for really, really awesome sex.

❥ *Oil-based Lubes and Massage Oils*

What makes a lubricant good for use inside the body (i.e., inside the vagina or anus)? First and foremost, it should not contain ANY oil or petroleum products in the ingredient list. Why not? Take a moment and reflect on your own hands when you're washing dishes or changing the oil. Once you get some oil on them, any water just beads up on your skin until you use an oil-cutting soap to clean up. It's pretty much the same deal for the vagina. If you put an *oil-based lube* (or lotion, or massage oil, etc.) into the vagina, it'll coat the walls of the vagina, covering the vaginal canal. Not a good plan, because the vagina cleans itself through transudation, where fluid comes through the walls of the vagina like an overfilled sponge. On the off chance that you happen to coat the walls with oil or oil-like substances, what winds up happening is that you're now preventing the vagina from going through its self-cleaning cycle. This results in it now being more susceptible to infections, and that's not how you want to treat one of your best pals. With the anus, there are some similar issues, plus your anus is connected to your intestines. Oil does not belong in them. Keep oil away from inside your body, and everyone is going to be a much happier camper.

So What Is It Good For?

Why might you want to use an oil-based lube? It's great for jacking off penises (though keep in mind that if you want to put that penis inside a vagina later, you're going to have to do some epic washing to make sure it's oil-free). Massage oils are great for, you guessed it, massages! Please note: oil-based lubes, oils, lotions, massage glides, and so on will break down latex, so if you'll be using latex gloves, dams, or condoms for safer sex, stay away from anything with oil to be extra safe.

Chapter

8

Backdoor Basics (Anal 101)

For some people, anal sex seems hot and sexy and is at the absolute top of their to-do list. For other people, it's beyond the bottom (pun intended) of that list, and sounds scary or gross. Of course, there are people who fall exactly in the middle on this topic. Anal sex of various types might be take it or leave it for them, or maybe they're interested in it but unsure about how to get started. Whichever camp you fall into, this chapter is all about hot backdoor action and should give you the information to decide whether some anal experimentation is for you.

Anal Sex Should Never Hurt

Not ever. The person receiving the penetration might feel some sort of pressure, but should not ever be in pain. Pain is your body's way of saying "STOP—something is wrong!" This means that if either of you are feeling pain at any point, you need to stop. Then you can reassess to see if there's something you can change to make it feel better and reengage, or hit pause on the posterior loving until you can make sure that you can proceed at a future date in a way that feels pleasurable for all involved. Remember, no pain = good. Pain = STOP NOW! Pain means that you're tearing delicate anal tissue, which is not good and can result in infections. No pain means that you're safe and good to go, and that your body is still doing well.

A Caveat

Anal sex is not the holy grail of sex. In fact, I hate to break it to you, but there's absolutely no magical type of sex that's going to make everything in your sex life ridiculously wonderful and life changing. Having happy and healthy anal sex may be amazing, it may be meh, or it may be "I don't ever want to do it again." Regardless of how it ends up for you and your partner, please make sure that you're making the choice to participate in anal sex and stimulation because YOU want to do it and experiment with it, not because you're feeling any pressure from a partner or even society about having anal sex. Anal sex under coercion is not and cannot be happy and healthy sex, and that's what this book is all about.

In this chapter, we're going to explore several topics that have to do with pleasuring the posterior:

X--- How do you get yourself into feeling up to getting down? The ways to relax, keep things clean, and chat up your lover.

X--- What's your anal MO? Do you want it slow and steady, are you ready for the grand finale, and what about strapping it on?

X--- Anal adventures additions: How to work in beads, plugs, and dildos.

Feeling Up to Getting Down

OK. You're ready. You want to learn more about your backdoor, the junk in your trunk, your badunkadunk. Heck, maybe you want to learn more about your partner's butt, tochas, or chocolate starfish. The brilliant thing is that everyone has an anus, so it's the great equalizer in the sex world. If you're feeling lots of pressure to be on the receiving end of sex, you can always turn things around (regardless of your partner's gender) and say, "Awesome! Anything you do to my butt, I want to do to your butt, too!" Sometimes this will be super exciting for them, or sometimes it might make them reconsider the amount of pressure they're putting on you to get it on from behind.

You're eager for more info. Of the following, which is your number one concern about anal sex, either as the giver or as the receiver?

➧ *Ways to Relax, page 131*

➧ *Keep Things Clean, page 134*

➧ *Chat up Your Lover, page 136*

➧ *Ways to Relax*

When people talk about being anal retentive, they're usually not talking about holding sex toys in their butt. Instead, we use the term *anal* to refer to people who are being uptight and super intense about things. To be honest, the anus can be like this in reality. Take a moment and tighten your anal sphincter. Now release it. Clearly, you have a conscious ability to tighten and loosen that sphincter, which is wonderful. In reality, your anus actually has two different sphincters, one internal and the other external. Only the external one is controlled consciously, while the internal one is controlled by your subconscious. This means that relaxation is a crucial part of getting ready for hot anal sex, because even if you THINK you're relaxed and ready to go, but internally are anxious and not ready for it to be happening, then you'll likely be able to relax one sphincter, but still feel uncomfortable with any penetration, because the other sphincter is like hellllll NO.

Don't Try to Check Out

How can you make sure that you're good and relaxed? The answer is NOT to get drunk or stoned before you're ready to get it on. Ditto on using anal numbing gels or creams. People tend to use anal numbing products (or to get drunk or high before anal sex) because they don't want to experience pain. However, if you're numb, it doesn't mean that the pain goes away; it just means that you're not experiencing it as it happens. This also means that the damage that you're causing to your anal tissue doesn't stop just because you can't feel it as it's happening. It's kind of like taking a Percocet and then hammering a nail through your hand … you're still putting the nail through your hand with or without the Percocet, but you just don't feel it or care as much when you're medicated. It's much better to get your body to relax enough (and use enough lube—CRUCIAL!) to have happy, healthy, pain-free anal sex that doesn't damage any of your body.

Bad Surprise

One way to feel more relaxed is to have some good conversation about anal sex with your partner before you do the deed. I cover this more specifically below, but surprise butt sex is a horrible idea in general. Surprising someone with anal stimulation can make them never want to try it ever again and can build up some epic distrust between people. Instead, making sure that you and your partner have talked about it, are both on board, and are both ready to communicate during it (and stop if it hurts) can go a long way to helping someone relax when they're thinking about having it.

Get Off Before You Go There

Another way to get ready and relaxed is for the person who will be receiving the anal penetration to have an orgasm (or multiple orgasms!) before any anal action starts to take place. Not only will this load up your whole system on fabulous endorphins that make everything feel that much better (think nomming on a whole bag of M&M's), but orgasms can help muscles to relax and in turn can help your whole body relax. Now things are feeling good, your body's relaxed, and you're much better positioned, in multiple ways, to be ready to go on an anal exploratory journey.

Get Handy Beforehand

Some people find that receiving a massage of any kind can help them feel more relaxed before getting in on the anal action. A back massage, a butt massage, even a foot massage can make you feel chill and relaxed, and ready to get some stimulation going. On the other hand, some people would prefer a nice spanking to get their butt all warmed up and ready for other sensations. Again, this is where communication is important. Make sure that you're both on the same page before you start spanking or lying down for a massage.

You can also get relaxed around your anal area by externally stimulating the area around your partner's anus—anyone can enjoy anal stimulation. Using lube to reduce drag, you can massage around the anal area, run your fingers over and around it, gently nibble on or bite the butt cheeks, and kiss around the whole area, until the muscles begin to get used to touch and stimulation. When it seems less intense and less scary, it helps the whole body, and both sphincters relax.

❧ *Keep Things Clean*

One of the top concerns about having sex that involves the butt is "What about the poop?!?!" To be honest, you touch poop every day, pretty much every time you touch a doorknob. I know, people are gross and don't wash their hands after using the bathroom, but it's true. You touch the bacteria from poop every day. Really, is that the worst thing that happens?

The Where of It

Here's the deal. Poop does not actually hang out in the bottom part of the anal canal and rectum near the anus. In fact, the anal canal/rectum is about five to ten inches long, and then bends into the sigmoid colon. Poop does hang out in the sigmoid colon, so unless you or your partner is actively feeling the need to poop (in which case, you or they should do so before you attempt having anal sex), you're not going to hit poop while you're putting things into the butt.

What about Residual Poop?
Despite popular belief, you don't need to use a douche or enema to properly clean out your anus. Now, if the idea of doing an enema feels amazing to you, then go for it, but dump out the chemicals that come in the prebought enema and just fill it with warm water, or even warm saltwater. Chemicals in your body are not a good idea and can cause irritation and reactions that increase pain and tearing, which I'm sure you don't want.

Good news! Rather than use an enema, you can head to your local drugstore and pick up a blue bulb syringe (sometimes referred to as "booger suckers"), fill that with warm water, and insert it into the anus (over the toilet), and just use it to rinse out your rectum. Any residual poop will be washed away.

Share a Shower
Of course, you can also both hop in the shower for some hot and soapy foreplay prior to anal playtime. Not only is the warm water a great way to help both of you (and all your muscles, including your anal muscles and sphincters) relax, but because you're showering together, you're both 100 percent reassured that both of you and all your genitals are clean and ready to go by the time you hop into bed. Use soap that is pH-balanced and moisturizing; you don't want to dry out your anal tissue right before you stick something in it.

Consider the Condom
The idea of safer sex might not have crossed your mind if you're in a monogamous, fluid-bound relationship (a relationship where you have both been tested and are OK sharing all your body fluids with each other). Keep in mind that using a condom, dams, or gloves can help keep things clean and tidy. If you use

a condom on a penis or dildo that's being used anally, you can just pull the condom off afterward. Then whatever was being used for penetration can then be used vaginally or orally (or using a condom can just save on cleanup time). Using gloves for manual stimulation helps solve the issue of long, sharp nails, and it also keeps your hands nice and clean. Black nitrile gloves are particularly great for this, as they don't show anything that might squick you out. Lastly, using dams (or even Saran Wrap) for analingus or oral-anal sex can help prevent the spread of anal bacteria, solve any issues you might have around the taste, and again, make for easy cleanup.

❥ *Chat up Your Lover*

OK. You think you're finally ready and raring to go about anal sex. Congrats! Now what? Sometimes, this can be one of those more difficult conversations to have with your partner. I mean, vaginal penetration of all sorts is already part of our usual sexual dialogue, and oral sex on both penises and vulvas is discussed in a ridiculous number of ways, including in songs and in movies. When it comes to butt sex, that seems like one of those more taboo conversational topics. How DO you ask someone to let you do them in the ass, or how do you request anal penetration for yourself?

Pick a Good Time to Talk

If it's something that you've never ever talked about or brought up in conversation before, then you're going to need to lay some groundwork, just like you would for any other new sexual activity (maybe check out the communication chapter for some additional suggestions in this realm). Just like with anal sex, you need to warm up the oven before you put anything in. Casually—NOT in the middle of sex or a fight (you'd be surprised at how frequently people decide that this is the best time to bring up a new sexual idea … it's not)—bring up a little bit of backdoor action. Perhaps you ask them if they've ever tried it or wanted to try it, or maybe you mention that your friend was talking about the film *Bend Over Boyfriend*, about women strapping it on and doing their boys in the butt. There are all sorts of ways to slide it into the conversation if you're not yet ready to be front and center with your interest in all things anal.

Your partner will likely react in one of three ways.

Way #1: They will be super-duper excited and ready to get it on. If this is the case, you need to pull back on the reins a little and let them know that you want to discuss things first. Make sure that you talk about who will be doing what to whom, what kind(s) of lube will be used, what toys (if any) will be involved, what safer sex will look like, who's in charge of the movement (the giver can be the person who pushes forward, or the receiver can ease gently back to let things in at their own speed), and so on. It's great that they're on the same page with you, but make sure you get in that crucial conversation to make sure that everyone's onboard with the same type of happy, healthy anal sex that you want to be having. It's possible that they may be even more gung ho about the booty loving than you are; it's absolutely OK to say that you're still pondering it, and that you just wanted to check with them before you made some serious plans around the anus.

Way #2: They're pretty meh about it. Not grossed out or offended, but not excited and down to play either. Maybe they have a few concerns, and I hope the rest of this chapter can help you address them. It's possible that they're worried that anal sex will hurt you or them, and you can be there to educate them about the plethora of ways to make sure that anal sex is painless and feels good. Perhaps they're concerned, like so many people, about the poop, and this is where you can step in and be super smart as you share all about the sigmoid colon and where the poop hangs out. Maybe they have some misinformation about things like anal numbing creams or think they need to be drunk to be done in the butt. You can set the record straight while making sure that they have the knowledge that they need. Once you're both on the same page, then you can move forward with the conversation about who's having what done to them (and by whom!), what toys and lubes need to be part of the picture, how safer sex will play a role, and so on.

Way #3: They pretty much, in their own language, give you the HEEEEEELLLLLL NO. There are lots and lots of reasons for this reaction. One reason might be a huge pile of misinformation, and responding in the way you would to Way #2 might help them feel more comfortable about even having this conversation (educating someone about happy and healthy anal sex is NOT ignoring their "no" or trying to change it — it's about making sure that they have good and accurate information). Another reason might be that they have trauma and/or triggers around anal sex. They might have had a bad experience with a partner, they might have had anal sex only because someone pressured them into it, or they might have had sexual assault involving anal sex (or had it happen to a friend or loved one). If this is the case, you need to be 100 percent supportive. You can always say that you're open to discussing the topic later, but that you'll let THEM bring it up if they ever feel comfortable … and then you need to put it down and walk away. Really, just drop it. If someone's experiencing a triggering or traumatic reaction to something, the best way to make it worse is to keep pushing the issue. Instead, offer them your support and validation, and let them guide the next steps of the conversation.

If their negative reaction is not because of those scenarios, you could ask them WHY they're so anti-anal, but again, make sure that they know you're validating their no. It may be a cultural thing or something they've never thought about, and you caught them off guard, or a multitude of other reasons. The best thing that you can do is to leave it alone. They now know that this is an activity that interests you and that they can bring it up in the future if their feelings change.

Learn All You Can

If you're in a neutral or positive place about anal, you might consider checking out an anal sex guidebook or some educational porn about anal (anything written by or directed by Tristan Taormino or Dr. Charlie Glickman is going to be particularly accurate and fabulous). You can read or watch the information together, or do it independently and then come together to … well … come together! Again, knowledge is power, and the more of it you have, the better your sexual experience will be. At the very least, make sure you're familiar with the rest of this section and have a lovely bottle of lube, and you should be hot to trot!

What's Your Anal MO?

You now have the basic 411 about anal action, and you're ready to figure out exactly how to make things happen in the posterior region.

Which of the following topics would you like to learn more about?

❯ *Slow and Steady*

Anal sex is a journey, not a goal. That may sound cheesy, but it's true. You have to make sure that the anus is ready and excited for play. It's not something to do in a hurry, or when you're stressed out, or when you're expecting your mother-in-law to show up in half an hour. The cliché that slow and steady wins the race is quite true; it's much better to begin at a slower pace and work your way up if everything is going well than it is to start out too speedy and end up needing to stop because it's uncomfortable or even painful.

Make Time for It

Because anal sex does require more time and sometimes more communication than other sexual activities (especially to begin with), it's important that you put aside time for anal. Foreplay looks like different things to different people, which is fine, but anal is going to require foreplay of some sort. It's not a wham, bam, thank you ma'am kind of activity, especially when you're just starting out. So take a moment and figure out what really turns each of you on, what actually gets your motor going. Is it a looooong make-out session? A little bit of playful spanking? Oral sex on one or both participants? Once you've figured out something that's going to raise the hotness quotient for both of you, get on it (perhaps literally). When both of you are already aroused, the endorphins coursing through your veins are likely to make everything else you do feel even better as you move forward. For many people, having an orgasm first before you even start to consider anal play can make all the sensations feel even better. For others, getting super turned on to *almost* getting to climax is the perfect place in their arousal cycle for them to be ready to begin anal play.

Back It Up

One great "trick" for anal sex is letting the person who's going to be receiving the anal stimulation take control of how much is going in, at what speed, and when. For example, if you're putting a smooth dildo into their butt, you can lube it up (for the love of all that's holy, please remember to use lots of lube!), place it gently at the opening (or even a centimeter or two inside the anus), and let them back into it, at their own pace. This way, they're 100 percent in control of how much they're taking in, letting them feel more comfortable and relaxed. You can also have them slip a scarf around the "giver's" waist, especially during intercourse with a penis or dildo, and have them pull their partner in close when they want more depth, and not pull when they need some time to relax into it.

Just the Tip Is Just Fine

Again, anal sex is an adventure with many stops along the way. Just because all you got in one night was the very tip of your pinky finger does NOT mean that you "failed" at having anal or that anything went wrong. Conversely, it sounds like you both communicated well to know what felt good, and when to stop, so that you'll both continue to have good feelings about anal sex and may want to continue having it. Moving slowly also allows a feeling of trust to develop between the partners, so that if you want to continue to move ahead with anal play in the future, you'll have a much easier time establishing trust, and for the receiver to know that the giver WILL in fact stop or slow down when asked. It's all about trust and communication, and making sure that everyone has a good time while exploring the sexual intricacies of the butt.

❧ *The Grand Finale*

At some point, the awesome anal adventure you're on has to end. However, like all types of sex, there's no one magic point that says "we're finished." Sure, you may choose to base it on either or both of you having an orgasm or climax of some sort, but frequently, it's not that easy. How do you know when to end anal, and what does it look like?

Semen Gets Around

If the person doing the penetrating has a penis, they may want to climax inside their partner. Make sure that if you're not using a condom, you have a discussion with your partner that this is hunky-dory with them and that you keep in mind the potential for semen cross-contamination with the vulva. If the receiver isn't on another form of birth control, leaking semen CAN come in contact with the vagina, and in some folks, could possibly make its way up to the cervix. If you have no plans to get pregnant, consider either using a condom for anal to be extra safe or maybe choosing to ejaculate elsewhere.

A Happy Ending

If the person receiving the anal penetration is able to climax from it (many people of all genders can in fact climax from anal stimulation), then this can be a part of the ending. They may want or need a little extra oomph from a vibrator, fingers, or a hand job during their arousal, so make sure you have some sex toys and/ or extra lube ready to go — trying to find the lube or your favorite vibe midsex is rarely fun and can sometimes lead to a sex fail as you fall off the bed trying to reach the Hitachi.

Something to keep in mind for fingers or penises inside the anus during orgasm is that many people's anal muscles clamp down VERY tightly as they climax. While this may feel good to some people, others might find it too intense for their body parts. Also, some people don't like to have anything inside their anus (or vagina, for that matter) as they climax, while others enjoy the feeling of being "full" during their orgasms. Again, this is communication that needs to happen, because you don't want one of you pulling out right as the other is climaxing if they like to have something inside, and you also don't want to be pushing in deeper during climax if they'd much rather you be out and done.

No One Way to Do It

Of course, as I've discussed, anal penetration is not the end-all, be-all of anal play. One of you might (with permission) stick your pinky into your partner's anus as they climax from other types of stimulation. You might pull anal beads out of your butt as your partner provides cunnilingus. There are all sorts of anal stimulation options, either by themselves or in conjunction with other types of sexual activity. And obviously, orgasms do not have to be part of all sexual play. If you want to provide analingus (oral-anal stimulation) to your partner because you both enjoy it, then go for it, and you can both decide when you've done enough. You can enjoy anal exploration as the main event, part of foreplay, or after other types of sex — whatever works best for you both.

Cleanup Is Key

Lastly, cleanup is important. If you used a condom over a penis or toy (or a glove over a hand, or a dam for oral stimulation), wrap it up in tissue or toilet paper, and toss it. Remember not to flush it, as it can damage and back up your sewer or septic system. If you weren't using a barrier, now is the time to do a warm water and soap wash of your hands, penises, toys, and so on. Remember that anal bacteria should never ever go into anyone's mouth or vulva—even if it's the same person whose anal bacteria it is. This can cause all sorts of infections and is no fun for anyone. If you used a toy anally without a barrier, you still need to wash it, and ideally, to sterilize it (boil it three to five minutes, put it on the top shelf of your dishwasher, or wipe it down with a 10 percent bleach solution and let it dry before washing it off again). If you can't sterilize it, make sure that both of you know that particular toys are only for anal use, and only for anal use in the person that it was always used in.

❥ *Strapping It On*

The idea of strapping it on, or having your partner strap it on, and having someone get done in the ass is incredibly appealing to you. Well, get in line, because anal sex with a harness and dildo is all the rage now across America. While anyone can strap it on and do anyone else in the butt (the anus is the great equalizer, right?), there's a growing trend of women (usually straight or bisexual women) strapping on a harness and dildo and giving it to their partners (usually straight men) in the butt. In fact, this sexual fad has become so popular that sex columnist Dan Savage decided to give it a special name: pegging. Ask anyone who works in a sex toy store—inquiries from straight couples about getting some strap-on action so that the woman can penetrate her man have grown exponentially over the past few years. Hot stuff.

As far as picking out the stuff that you need to strap it on (usually a harness and a dildo, unless you decide to go the route of the double dildo), check out the couples' toys section in chapter 7, which goes into excruciating detail about how to pick out the perfect dildo and harness combo for you and your partner's needs. Once you've procured these wondrous sex toys, it's time to figure out how to make the magic happen.

Who Puts What Where
First, whoever's going to be strapping it on (which could be both of you, if that's what gets you going) should take a moment to try on the whole strap-on contraption (harness AND dildo) before it's time to get down and dirty. That gives them the chance to figure out which strap goes where, what needs to be tightened, and where they feel comfortable having the dildo sit on their pelvis. Walk around a little—cock confidence is something gained by spending a little time getting comfortable, and eventually confident, wearing this sexy and exciting new getup.

LUBE
Next, you're going to need lube. I know, I've said it before and I'll say it again, but lube is love folks, ESPECIALLY with anal action and ESPECIALLY with sex toys. Silicone toys (really, most sex toy materials) have a lot more drag than just skin on skin, so lube is crucial for optimizing your sexual experience.

Missteps Happen
Sometimes, while you're wearing a harness and dildo and penetrating your partner, the dildo will fall out. It's OK; it happens

with attached penises too, far more often than you might expect. The issue is that during strap-on action, you might not notice that you've fallen out (because you can't feel your partner through the dildo). Don't panic; just make sure you communicate with your partner and have them let you know if you happen to miss. If they don't tell you, and you don't know, you might have a few awkward moments of hip thrusting into nothing, but once you figure it out, pop it (gently) back in, and you'll be good to go again. Laugh it off, get some more endorphins flowing in your system, and you're back in the saddle.

Want more instruction? There are multiple guides to strap-on sex that'll give you a little bit more of an in-depth (ha-ha) look into strap-on play. Also, the DVD of *Bend Over Boyfriend* is basically a pegging 101 film. Starring the sex educator Carol Queen, this film showcases a variety of male-female couples, where the woman is strapping it on and giving everything she's got to her male partner. It offers some communication hints, as well as excellent tips and techniques to making sure your pegging (or general strap-on) experience is truly as fabulous as it can possibly be.

Anal Adventures Additions: Beads, Plugs, and Others

The world is almost always more fun when you add some toys to the table. If you or your partner (or even both of you) enjoy receiving anal stimulation of the manual sort, then using an anal-friendly dildo (with or without a vibrator), butt beads, or an anal plug (again, with or without a vibrator) can provide fabulous sensation as part of foreplay, during a non-anal sexual activity, or of course, as the main course.

Remember that everyone has an anus—it's the great equalizer! Either one or both partners can enjoy anal stimulation as part of sex, and it can help to pleasure one partner while they're concentrating on giving pleasure to the other.

Crucial Words of Caution

I've said it before and I'll say it again! You ALWAYS need to use some type of lubricant when working with the anus (internally or even externally), and that goes double for when you're using anal safe-sex toys, because they can create extra drag. Also, anything that you're going to stick in the butt needs to have a flanged base. What is that? This means that the base is wider than the rest of the toy. Any sex toy (vibes, dildos, Kegel balls, etc.) without a base should never ever, EVER be put in the butt. Ever. Of course, you should always warm up the anus for a good bit before putting a toy inside.

Which of the following seems like something fun and exciting to put in your backdoor?

- ❥ *Butt Beads Galore! page 147*
- ❥ *Anal Plugs to Have and to Hold, page 149*
- ❥ *Something With a Little More In and Out, page 150*

❥ Butt Beads Galore!

Butt beads are meant to be placed in one at a time, and can be gently pulled out during or right around the time of orgasm. They're a great way to slowly warm up your butt to the idea of having something in it, and can be a great introduction to anal play. Flexi Felix from Fun Factory is my favorite recommendation in this category, but lots of companies offer good-quality silicone anal beads. Please make sure that they're silicone—anything going into your ass needs to be made of a material that can be sterilized, so plastic just won't cut it.

What's Up with Butt Beads

Despite the image of a string of beads like a necklace that might pop into your mind when you hear "beads," that's not generally what butt beads look like. In fact, you don't want to use any sort of beads attached by a string. Not only can the string get covered in bacteria, but it can also rot and break (and it'll get lost in your ass).

Good butt beads are a series of connected medium- to large-sized beads, sometimes starting with a small bead and increasing in size. They may be piled up right on top of the other, or there may be thin lengths between the beads covered with silicone. Either way, they should all be one continuous piece of material.

How Do You Use Anal Beads?

You want to just put in one bead at a time, making sure that it's well lubricated. If one bead feels good, then you can move on to the next one, adding as many as feel good or comfortable to you at that point. Once everything you want is in, you can do anything you want. You may enjoy leaving them in while you provide other forms of stimulation to yourself or your partner, or you can gently pull them out. Many people enjoy having them removed at the point of orgasm. Just remember not to pull them out lawn-mower style. Not only would that be incredibly uncomfortable for the ass that they were being pulled from, but extra lube might come swinging out with it, and that's a whole new kind of cleanup that you probably weren't planning for.

❧ *Anal Plugs to Have and to Hold*

A butt plug or anal plug (vibrating or not) is meant to be gently worked into the anus, and then just stay in during whatever activity is taking place. You can use it to have that fun, full feeling during other types of sex play, or you can wear it in advance of anal penetration to get your butt used to having something inside it.

What They're Good for, and What They Aren't

Contrary to some people's beliefs, butt plugs aren't meant to be pulled or pushed in and out of the ass. Because the anal sphincters close around the neck to hold it in place, trying to use it like a dildo can be incredibly uncomfortable for the person wearing the plug. Just lube it up nicely and then gently slide it in, allowing the body to close around it. If the person wearing it also happens to have a vagina, they might enjoy receiving penetration while wearing a plug, although definitely start on the milder side before working your way into a frenzy to best gauge how it feels to them. If the wearer of the butt plug has a penis, a blow job while wearing an anal plug can feel particularly nice (as can cunnilingus on a vulva). Basically, other than sticking additional things in the butt, you can do pretty much anything you want while wearing a butt plug, including running errands, giving a lecture, or running on the treadmill. Make it work for you!

If you or your partner is working your way up to being penetrated in the butt with a penis or dildo, wearing an anal plug beforehand can help you out. It allows your anal muscles to relax around the plug while gently preparing both the muscles and sphincter for whatever might be coming their way. You can take it out before penetration, re-lube, and then, starting slowly, go for the bigger item. Plus, you can always use wearing a butt plug as a sign that you're raring to go for some butt sex. Just bend over so that the other person can see it, and it'll act like a signal flag, waving them on in to the anal area!

What to Look For

While many butt plugs are made of medical grade silicone (both Tantus and Vixen Creations have fabulous options), there are also those created out of other sterilizable materials that can be fun in many ways. Crystal Delights makes an absolutely beautiful glass butt plug that has a Swarovski crystal on its base, so you can really bling your thing, if that's what you like. Njoy has come out with a beautiful stainless steel metal plug in multiple sizes: classy, unbreakable, and also able to be sterilized. Recently, corian has come onto the market as a nonporous material that's marketed as sterilizable, and I've seen plugs made out of this as well.

❥ *Something with a Little More In and Out*

An anal dildo is meant more to go in and out (either partner can operate this), either handheld or attached to a harness as part of fabulous strap-on sex. Most of these dildos are going to be on the slimmer side, a little thinner than other dildos, and most people prefer smoother-feeling dildos for anal play, although if you or your partner prefer more of the nubs and ridge action, I say go for it. Because you want something that you can sterilize, you're going to want to stick with silicone, glass, metal, and ceramic. These toys can be boiled, dishwashed, or wiped down with a 10 percent bleach solution (allow it to dry, and then wash it off again) after use, even if you're using it in the same person. Anal bacteria should never go into the vagina or mouth, even if it's the same person using the toy in their own anus.

Don't Forget the Flange

Don't forget that anything you put in your anus, including dildos, should have a wide (flanged) base, making it safe for anal use without the fear of anything getting lost. If a dildo is designed to fit in a harness for strap-on play, then you can be sure it's also safe for anal use. If you're not sure whether the base is going to be big enough for safety, then likely it's not. Find a different toy.

Fun for All!

You can use anal dildos on yourself or on your partner, or have your partner use them on you. If you want, you can just penetrate with it while holding it, or you can add in other fun sensations like cock rings, vibrators, and so on. Of course, you also have the wonderful opportunity of getting a good silicone dildo and combining it with an awesome harness, and either strapping it on and giving it to your partner, or having them strap it on and go to town on you. Just make sure the receiver is adequately lubed, and to either re-lube (if using silicone lube) or add water to re-activate water-based lube to keep things nice and wet throughout the whole sexual process.

Chapter

G Is for G-spot and Female Ejaculation

Perhaps you've heard of this sometimes secretive and perhaps mysterious spot known as the G-spot. You want to know more about it, how to stimulate it, where it is, what it does, and whether it's worth all the hype. In this chapter you'll learn all the goodness about:

X--- G-spots: Delving into the cave of wonders, discovering the G, and the expertise about the G both then and now.

X--- Female Ejaculation: Whether you're like the Sahara or Old Faithful, find out what it's all about how to make it happen.

Are You a G-spot Spelunker?

As we delve into the wonderful world of the G-spot, you should decide what basic information you want. Which topic is of most interest to you?

❥ *Entering the Cave of Wonders*

There are more nicknames for *vagina* than you can shake a dildo at, but even so, sadly, lots of people know almost nothing of the anatomy of the vulva and vagina. Lots of people don't even know what the word *vulva* means. Luckily, I'm going to drop some knowledge on you so that you'll be much better equipped to get some vulvar and vaginal loving going on.

Va-Va-Va-Vulva

Let's start with the vulva. Basically, the vulva is the whole enchilada, and the vagina is the delicious filling inside. The vulva encompasses the mons pubis (a.k.a. the mound of venus, or the pubic bone), the outer labia, the inner labia, the clitoris, the clitoral hood, the urethra, and the vagina. I use the terms *inner lips* and *outer lips*, because they can be different sizes (so labia majora and labia minora are inaccurate terms)—the big difference is that the outer labia naturally have hair and the inner lips don't. What you do with your pubic hair is entirely up to you—you can shave it, wax it, braid it, dye it, trim it, leave it. Just don't let anyone else tell you the right or wrong way to have pubic hair, because there isn't one. It's all up to the person whose pubic hair it is.

Love That Clitoris!

Above the two sets of lips is the clitoral glans (the very tip of the clitoris) and the clitoral hood. The hood's entire purpose is to act like a large eyelid for the clitoris, protecting it during normal activities so that it doesn't get rubbed or bruised when you're walking to class or running on the elliptical. As you get more and more aroused, it pulls back, allowing access to the clitoris itself. (For some women, the hood comes back down again about thirty to sixty seconds before orgasm. Of course, this can be super annoying to partners who think they're doing something wrong and decide to switch up their strokes right before climax. If this happens, just let them know to keep doing what they're doing, and not to stop.) The clitoral glans is the head of the clitoris, just like the glans of the penis is the head of the penis. The actual clitoris (get ready for this) is about three to six inches long. Yup. It's shaped like a wishbone, and the legs of the clitoris run underneath the inner labia. This is one of the many reasons it feels good to stimulate the inner labia, and it's also why many women prefer girth rather than length, because the girthier the fingers, toys, penises, and so on are, the better they stimulate the clitoris's long legs as they go in and out. Amazing, right?

Your Urethra

Right between the clitoral glans/hood and the vaginal opening is the urethra. This is indeed where urine comes out from the bladder, but it's also where ejaculatory fluid can come out. No, it's NOT pee. Studies have found that ejaculatory fluid in women contains little to no urea, the main ingredient found in urine. Instead, it comes from the Skene's glands, which are inside the urethra, but not connected at all to the bladder. Check out the section on ejaculation for more info.

The Ins and Outs of the Vagina

Last, but certainly not least, we have the vagina and vaginal canal. The vaginal canal runs from the vaginal opening all the way to the cervix, which is kind of like the cap at the end of the vagina. The depth of an "average" vagina is five to seven inches, which is why the whole conversation about women wanting foot-long penises is kind of silly, since most women's vaginas aren't long enough to take insertables of that length.

Vaginas grow slightly in length and in width as they get turned on, and of course, can also stretch out if they're giving birth. The cervix is the end of the vagina and has a tiny opening called the os, which lets menstrual blood through and dilates during birth. You cannot actually lose anything in the vagina—if you get worried about it, just reach your fingers in (or have your partner reach their fingers in), and you can get out errant condoms, tampons, sex toys, Kegel balls, and so on. Some people like having their cervix touched and massaged because it feels sexy to them, but other people don't, and touching the cervix can cause cramping in some people. Make sure you communicate how you feel about it to your partner so that they don't touch you in a way that'll wind up not feeling good.

The Rest of the Neighborhood

Then there's the area between the vaginal opening and the anus. Different people call this area different names, from the 'tain't (because it 'tain't the vagina and it 'tain't the anus) to no-man's-land, to the special spot. The official scientific name for this area is the perineum, and for many people (of all sexes and genders), it can feel really good to rub, because there are many nerve endings running underneath that area.

❧ *Discovering the G*

The G-spot has a rap as one of the most elusive and hard-to-find pleasure areas on the female body. Now, I'm not saying that looking for it is as easy as hunting for the nose on your partner's face, but it also doesn't require an excessive amount of vaginal spelunking to find it.

G Marks the Spot

While not one body is normal or "average," the G-spot can usually be found about one to three inches into the vagina on the top (anterior) wall (on the same side of the body as the belly button). While the vagina is textured overall, the G-spot is a special area that engorges with blood as the person becomes aroused. When it's engorged, it feels a bit more three-dimensional than the rest of the wall. It's about the size of a quarter, give or take a little. People frequently compare it to feeling like the shell of a walnut, but I've never met a vaginal canal that feels hard like a walnut. Instead, run your tongue along the roof of your mouth—that texture up there is much more similar to the texture of the G-spot than any shelled nut.

G Is Ghost?

The biggest challenge in finding the G-spot is that it isn't always there. Now, if you go to sleep with a pinky finger, you wake up with a pinky finger. And your kneecaps usually don't wander off in the middle of the night. However, the G-spot comes into existence only when you're turned on and blood rushes to your genitals, engorging the G-spot. This means that if you or your partner decides to go hunting for it out of boredom, or solely for the goal of finding the G-spot, you might have some issues in finding it. Of course, if you make your G-spot exploration part of foreplay, the main event, or a journey to be undertaken after a few orgasms, you're much more likely to have success.

G Is Not for Grail

A reminder: The G-spot, while awesome, is not the holy grail of sex. Many women love receiving G-spot stimulation, but if you and your partner don't already click, G-spot stimulation is not going to solve the issues you already have. It's not an alternative solution to all other types of sex—you still will need to communicate with your partner about your wants and needs. Some people find that they love G-spot stimulation, others see it as a fun adventure or welcome addition to other types of sex, some feel that it's a take it or leave it kind of thing, and some couldn't care less. Whichever way you feel about your G-spot and G-spot stimulation is absolutely OK.

A Hard Solo Expedition

Most people have trouble stimulating their own G-spot by themselves, especially without the use of a toy. A lot of people don't have the flexibility to reach down, put their fingers into their own vagina, and still have enough length left to find their G-spot. If you're looking for the G-spot on your own, it could be helpful to use a toy. The best toys for G-spot stimulation are those that are longer (an insertable style of toy) and are a harder material (either metal, glass, ceramic, or a firmer silicone/silicone-covered vibrator) with a curved end, or ball on the end. The firmness allows you to push up into the G-spot without it moving away, and the curve helps find the G-spot.

Doing It by Hand

If someone's trying to find the G-spot with their fingers, a great way to explore is to have the possessor of the G-spot lying on her back, with her legs spread and bent at the knee. If the explorer slides their fingers into the vagina, and curves them up, making a "come hither" or "coochie coochie coo" motion, they should be able to slide them in both deeper and shallower to find the G-spot.

Knowing You've Arrived

How do you know when you've found the G-spot? When either you or a partner presses down on your G-spot, you'll likely feel the sensation that you have to pee. Because of this, I highly recommend peeing before you hop into bed for your G-spot exploration, so that you're not worried about having to pee (if you just went to the bathroom, it's unlikely that you'll have to go again right away—this can be super useful in allaying your fear that you might accidentally pee). The longer you press on or stimulate the G-spot, the "have to pee" sensation should dissipate, and eventually, it should just feel good and pleasurable. Again, the amount of pleasure will vary from person to person—for some people, it might feel like a deep, internal pleasure button, but for others, it might be more of a lesser or dilute pleasure that feels good, but doesn't feel absolutely amazing when pressed.

Don't Fall for G Gimmicks

A variety of gels and creams claim to increase G-spot stimulation and engorgement. There is also G-spot enhancement surgery that claims to add fluid to further engorge your G-spot. Honestly, most of these gels and surgeries are gimmicks, designed to encourage women to feel anxious about their sexual ability and sexual performance. You don't need any type of plastic surgery to enhance your G-spot or any of your sexual anatomy—good communication about what feels good and what doesn't is more than enough to ensure that you have a happy, healthy sex life.

Kegels Are the Key to G-spot Os

Are you interested in having deeper, stronger, and more intense orgasms with vaginal and G-spot stimulation? Try working out your vagina, and I'm not talking about any fancy equipment that you can find only at the gym. I'm talking about exercising your Kegel and PC muscles.

It's easy—you've probably done it before. Let's do it together. Pretend that you're peeing (but don't actually do it right now). Take a moment to squeeze your muscles in like you're trying to stop the flow of your pee (if needed, you definitely could try it while peeing if you need that support in finding your PC muscles, but make sure to not stop the flow of your urine very often—it's not good for your body and can lead to other health issues). SQUEEEEEEZE in. Now, push out, like you're peeing. Squeeze in again. Keep it going—this is the simplest and easiest way to work out your Kegel muscles! To continue this exercise, you have lots of options; try squeezing them in and holding for about five to ten seconds, then let out the muscles. You can also attempt to pulse them in and out for thirty seconds, and then take a break. Basically, anything that you can do with this muscle group can help work it out. As with any other muscle group in your body, you have to start out slowly and build your muscles.

As you continue to work them out for a while, you can tighten and hold your muscles for a longer period. You don't have to do this all by yourself—it can also be fabulous to do this type of workout while you have a hand/penis/toy inside you. If you need a little extra help, try Kegel balls (meant to be worn while you walk around, to help you with your exercises), Kegelcisors, or Kegel barbells, which are further discussed in the sex toy section.

Bonus Benefits of Strong Kegel Muscles

What good are super-strong PC or Kegel muscles? These pelvic floor muscles can help you to have more intense orgasms, and having stronger vaginal muscles can help support multiple orgasms, as well as make it more possible to have female ejaculation. It's not possible for most women to ejaculate when they have weak PC muscles, so if learning to ejaculate sounds like something fun to you, you'll want to start building up those muscles now, to ensure your Kegels are nice and strong for when you decide to explore ejaculation.

The Destination Can Be in the Journey

Like other types of sex, G-spot exploration is a bit of a journey. You can discover it in various ways, and add G-spot stimulation to other activities, or make your G-spot adventure the highlight of playtime. Whatever works best for you and your partner, and feels good to you, is the best way to enjoy your particular G-spot. Something to keep in mind is that your sensitivity on your G-spot may change throughout your menstrual cycle. This is something to think about if you notice changes in how you feel, and to communicate to your partner or partners.

❥ *G-spot Experts—Then and Now*

Some of the first conversation around the G-spot started back in the seventeenth century (no, this is not just some random, modern phenomena) when a physician from the Netherlands (Dr. Graaf) wrote about female ejaculation and an area of pleasure on the anterior wall of the vagina that may cause pleasure. Of course, since this was pretty early in the ongoing conversation about female sexual pleasure (which lots of people have spent centuries debating whether or not it exists), no one took him seriously. The ball was dropped until the 1940s, when Dr. Gräfenberg (for whom the G-spot was later named) wound up doing research on urethral stimulation and discovered this pleasure zone in the majority of his female research subjects. While he didn't write a significant amount on the G-spot, his few remarks on the area as an erotic zone led to him becoming known as the father of the G-spot, and of course, having it named after him.

Modern Research
There was no real movement on the G-spot debate within the scientific community for another few decades (although women who had discovered their own G-spots were of course already well versed on the matter) until a team of researchers in the 1980s, lead by Beverly Whipple and Alice Kahn Ladas, published a book about their research on the G-spot (the book was called *The G Spot and Other Recent Discoveries about Human Sexuality*, and is still for sale today, if you'd like a little light reading). Like all previous discussions on the G-spot, this was received both well and with many challenges. Many people, including doctors and scientists, continue to believe that the G-spot doesn't in fact exist, contrary to much research and empirical evidence to the contrary.

There's Always Some Naysayers
Back in 2010 or so, a British study came out, saying that it was definitive that the G-spot, in fact, didn't exist. Never mind the millions of women from around the world who claimed that they had found their G-spot and enjoyed G-spot stimulation. Never mind the millions of partners of women who claimed that they had felt and stimulated G-spots in their partners. No, this study said it actually didn't exist. Then, it later turned out that this study

had no actual hands-on research and was done via surveys instead of hands-on research. Because a significant number of women had answered that they didn't think they had a G-spot, or had not been able to find their G-spot, the scientists concluded that the G-spot didn't exist. Many women read this study and were subsequently confused, as they had experienced the G-spot and were now being told that it simply didn't exist. However, as more details of the study came to light, it was realized that this was not the most scientifically accurate way to prove or disprove the existence of a body part, and most people have moved on from it since it was released.

It's quite hard to study the G-spot scientifically. Unlike every single other body part on anybody of any sex or gender, the G-spot doesn't always exist. It engorges with fluid only when the owner of said G-spot is aroused. Because of this, the G-spot is not found on cadavers studied in medical communities, and it's incredibly difficult to study in a lab setting. Why? Because unless the subject has a medical fetish and is aroused by being put in a gynecological chair while having her vagina subjected to probes and prodding, the G-spot is not going to come out and play with researchers. In fact, the most successful studies done on both the G-spot and female ejaculation have been conducted by having the research subjects stimulate themselves in ways that are incredibly arousing to them (including, in some studies, to the point of orgasm or climax). Studying these participants' vaginas after they've already experienced arousal makes it much easier to find and therefore demonstrate the real-life existence of the G-spot.

Ejaculation: Not Just for Penises Anymore (or Ever)!

All right, folks. We've covered the basics of the G-spot. Great! Now, lots of people want to know about the squirting, gushing, and so on that's so frequently associated with the G-spot.

Which of these best represents your own experience with ejaculation from your own body?

- ❥ *The Sahara, page 163*
- ❥ *A Riveting River, page 166*
- ❥ *Old Faithful, page 168*

❥ *The Sahara*

You've never ejaculated before and are starting to wonder what the big deal is, or maybe you're frustrated that you've never quite been able to gush to your wishes. To that, I say that ejaculation can be a bit of a Pandora's box. Yes, it's incredibly fun and fabulous, but most people have found that once they get started ejaculating, they can't stop. Once the floodgates have opened, there's not much of a way to stop the flow or, sometimes, even control it at all. That said, if you're willing to do the extra laundry of towels that may pile up with ejaculation, then feel free to keep on reading.

What It Is and Isn't

One of the important things to learn about this ejaculatory fluid that comes forth from the vagina? IT IS NOT PEE. Let's put that in different words: this ejaculatory fluid is not urine, it's not pee, and it doesn't contain urea like pee or urine does. Of course, there's absolutely nothing wrong with urine at all (interestingly enough, when urine comes out of your body, it's 100 percent sterile, which is more than you can say for saliva), but in case you were worried about it, along with millions of other people, you can take comfort in the fact that you now know that it's not pee, even though it comes out of the urethra.

Just so you know, ejaculate is created in the Skene's glands (as opposed to the bladder, which is where urine is created), and if the G-spot is fully aroused and engorged through stimulation, these glands can sometimes release ejaculatory fluid through the urethra. There's no perfect equation for how to make ejaculation happen—in fact, it can happen at the same time as an orgasm, it can happen without an orgasm happening, and of course, orgasms can happen without ejaculation being part of the equation. All of these are completely normal and, of course, fun and sexy.

Drops or Buckets, It's All Good

The amount of ejaculate that is, well, ejaculated, can vary between a few drops and the better part of half a cup. It all depends on the person doing the ejaculating, her hydration level (your body isn't going to expel fluid if it's worried about being dehydrated), how her body works, and many other factors. As with vaginal lubrication, the amount of ejaculate has no correlation to how aroused the person is. Period.

Preparing for the Flood

If you or your partner turns out to be an ejaculator, let's first talk about preparing for the flood. You can put down some extra towels on the bed before things start getting hot and heavy, or you can buy a few "puppy pads" at the grocery or pet store to place under your bodies (if you don't want to be doing heaps of laundry)—they're plastic on one side, absorbent on the other, so that you don't have to worry about any leakage. Towels and puppy pads are also great for sex during your period—easy to clean up and a fun way to relieve cramps!

Good Things Take Time

As far as the actual ejaculation itself, remember that time, patience, and not making anything a goal are all parts of trying something new, and working on ejaculation is not expectation. Oftentimes, people find it easier to work on ejaculation after they've already had an orgasm, so that they're not focusing on whether or not to climax, and so that the G-spot is already engorged with blood because it's so aroused. Consider climaxing from your favorite method of stimulation first and then start your ejaculation journey.

Getting There Is Great!

Have yourself or your partner stimulate your G-spot with either fingers or toys (most people learn to ejaculate this way, rather than in the middle of intercourse with a penis or dildo). Breathe into it, and as you feel that "need to pee" sensation, push out, like you're going to pee. If you're really worried about the potential for pee, just make sure that you pee before you get started, so that you know that your bladder is empty and you're good to go. If you hold in your Kegel muscles, like you do in your Kegel or PC muscle exercises, that'll prevent ejaculation, because everything's clamped down. Most people have to learn how to press their vaginal floor muscles out instead of in before they can ejaculate. Press out and add some clitoral stimulation (fingers, a vibrator, or a mouth) while you or your partner continues to stimulate your G-spot with a firm pressure, moving in and out. It's fine if you don't ejaculate the first time, or every time. Again, this is something that's much more of a journey than just a goal, and you should make sure you get to enjoy every step of the way there.

Not for Everyone

Lastly, not everyone ejaculates. Yes, every woman has a G-spot, but it may not be something she finds particularly arousing, and her body may choose not to be the type of body that ejaculates. Just because you or your partner is unable to ejaculate doesn't mean that there's anything wrong with you or that you're not having extremely hot and pleasurable sex. It also doesn't mean that you'll never be able to ejaculate. Lots of people try for years to learn how to ejaculate, and nothing ever happens. Then a few years, or a few partners, down the road? Kazaam! They're suddenly free flowing like a magnificent stream, ejaculating here, there, and everywhere. Whether you ejaculate has nothing to do with how pleasurable sex is or whether you're "doing it right" (remembering that there's in fact no way to have sex the "right" way)—as long as you and your partner(s) are enjoying yourselves, that's all that matters.

❧ *A Riveting River*

So you've already discovered much of the magic that makes up the mystical world of ejaculation, but perhaps you're not sure what's really happening or you just want more info on what's going on below the belt.

Making a Map to the River

Maybe you ejaculated once with one partner, or while experimenting on your own, and you're looking to make it happen again.

Think for a moment about the situation when your ejaculatory explosion took place. Who was it with? What toys (or body parts) were you using? Had you already had an orgasm before you started the G-spot stimulation, or did you go straight into playing with that special zone? Were you relaxed or stressed? Pressing out or tightening your vaginal muscles?

Once you've figured out what it took in the past to get to a level of ejaculatory adventures, you can work to re-create it. Just remember that the more pressure you place on any activity, to try and reach any goal, the less likely it is that you'll achieve it. Your body gets stressed out when you're too focused on something, preventing it from relaxing enough to get to the point where you CAN ejaculate again. It's the body's catch-22.

If you're trying things out with your partner, make sure you clue them in to your plans. Trying and trying without them knowing what's going on might be a little awkward. Once you let them in on it, consider fun ways that you can experiment together. Who knows? They might even have some creative new suggestions that get you exactly where you want to go.

Make It Rain!

Let's talk liquids, too. If you're dehydrated, or even just semi-hydrated, it makes it hard for your body to release extra fluid in a superfluous manner, like ejaculation tends to be. Without adequate hydration, your body saves all the existing fluid to run your systems. If you're interested in the prospect of ejaculating, make sure to take a couple of extra ounces of H2O before you slip between the sheets so your body knows you're good to go.

❧ *Old Faithful*

You, like a certain geyser in Yellowstone National Park, go off with alarming clockwork regularity. Your G-spot is touched and out come the rushing waters. Mazel tov—you've certainly hit the jackpot of ejaculation.

Some Extras You Might Appreciate

So why is there a section for you? Let's talk about some ways to make ejaculating less intrusive. How many towels do you go through regularly to prevent a "wet spot" of gargantuan proportions on the bed? You may want to consider investing in a miracle invention from Liberator (yes, the same company that makes all that brilliant sex furniture) called the Fascinator Throe, and yes, it's spelled that way.

The Throe is truly one of the best creations of the twenty-first century, especially for those of us who squirt and gush like champions. What is it? It looks like a throw blanket (hence the name), but has two different textures—one side is a soft microfiber or microsuede, and the other side is a silky satin. Sounds nice, but what does it have to do with ejaculation? The brilliance of the Throe is that it's waterproof in the middle, meaning that if you're lying on it when the waters come, the blanket catches all of them, and doesn't let them drip through to the other side. Instead, you just fold up or scrunch up the Throe, toss it aside, cuddle and/or sleep, and then later you throw the whole thing into the wash. Absolutely brilliant! It comes in various colors and prints, so that you can make it match your bedroom. It's also great for traveling, so you don't get ejaculate all over the couch in the hotel or on your partner's bed the first or second time you're getting it on (before they invest in more towels).

Some Contest, It's the Best!
Plus, you can have a lot of fun with this sexual talent of yours. Masturbate-a-thons around the country (to celebrate May being National Masturbation Month) have lots of games and contests around ejaculatory fluid—who can squirt the farthest, who ejaculates the most fluid, and so on. While you may not be ready to travel to one of these events or compete in public, you could certainly have some competitions against yourself, changing the variables (what type of stimulation, how much liquid you imbibe beforehand, etc.) to figure out what helps you to ejaculate the farthest and the most. You can also try changing the color of the ejaculate by eating beets (or drinking juiced beets), taking B-12 vitamins, and more. If you want to have fun with having the ejaculatory ability you have, then go for it.

Be Proud of Your Plenty
Sadly, many women with the natural ability to ejaculate (or those who have trained themselves to ejaculate through experiment and exploration) have been shamed by friends, partners, and even doctors for this ability. To me, this is heartbreaking. No one should be made to feel less than amazing for anything they can do with their body. In fact, there are many people out there who have been trying for years to learn how to ejaculate and simply have not been able to, a great example of how the grass truly is greener on the other side. Lots of potential partners find ejaculation to be exciting and interesting to watch, and would probably be thrilled to be partnered with someone who can ejaculate. So if you're one of those people who's been told anything negative about your outstanding ability, leave all that behind in the dust and emerge as someone proud of your sexual talent, ready to show the world whether you're a squirter, a gusher, or just someone who likes to ejaculate.

Chapter

10

Naughty Can Be Nice (Kink 101)

It's time to talk about getting a bit kinky up in here. Perhaps you love Rihanna's "Whips and Chains" song or found that *Fifty Shades of Grey* made you feel wet between your legs. Regardless of how you discovered your interest in the world of kink or BDSM, welcome!

What does BDSM even mean? It stands for three acronyms within four letters: bondage and discipline, domination and submission, and sadism and masochism. People who feel that they're kinky can be into any of these things, all of these things, or some combination. Maybe you just have some fantasies of tying your lover to the bed or of getting a spanking for being such a naughty girl. On the other hand, maybe you're ready to invest in turning your bedroom into your own dungeon or going out and playing in your local kink community. As long as everything is consensual, anything and everything under the sun is absolutely A-OK.

In this chapter, we're going to cover the three basic areas of kink and BDSM:

X--- Power play: Are you deliciously dominant, sweetly submissive, or do you like to switch it up?

X--- A little impact with your pleasure: Do you want spankings, floggings, or caning and crops?

X--- Bound by love: When it comes to getting tied up, do you want silky scarves, captivating cuffs, or rocking ropes?

Power Play

First, let's talk about power, and see if there's some hot and sexy power play evident in your fantasies about kink. Of the following options, which do you identify with the most?

❥ *Deliciously Dominant, page 171*

❥ *Sweetly Submissive, page 174*

❥ *A Sexy Switch, page 176*

❥ *Deliciously Dominant*
You think to yourself about how incredibly sexy it would be to be in total control of someone, with your lover obeying your commands or taking their rightful place at your feet. Maybe

the idea of a collar around your partner's neck gets your engine going, or perhaps it's the sound of the words "Yes, Ma'am" that truly get your panties in a twist. You want to have sexual control of the situation and are ready to make dominance your middle name.

Where the Power Lies

Wanting to be in charge in the bedroom does not always equate to wanting to be in charge with the rest of your life. Lots of people switch to the opposite of their day-to-day roles. Powerful lawyers and CEOs want to be submissive, while those who take orders as part of their day job may wind up craving control when their clothes come off. Additionally, wanting to be in a dominant role in a sexual relationship doesn't mean that you're a controlling jerk—people who are being dominant with their partners need to be more attuned to their partner's feelings and need more than your average run-of-the-mill person, because being dominant is about BOTH of you enjoying the power play and not just being mean to or dominating someone else.

What Can Dominance Look Like in a Relationship?

It can be as simple as telling your partner to call you Miss, Ma'am, Mistress, Goddess, Oh Beautiful One, and so forth. You can make this the rule for all sexual experiences, or maybe just when you're wearing your "dominant" outfit, or on the second Thursday of every month. While some people integrate power play into their entire relationship, or even most of their sexual experiences, many others enjoy power play as just something exciting to do now and then. You might think of a title to use for your partner when they take on the submissive role—boy/girl, slave, lowly one, or you might not want to use a title at all. It's up to you!

Safety Word First

Something that's incredibly important when you play with power, especially if you want someone to be able to say no, and it not actually MEAN no (like if you're tickling someone or continually bringing them to orgasm, and they want to be able to say, "No, no, no, I can't take any more, STOP!" without you actually stopping), is to come up with something called a safeword. This concept has been discussed more and more in mainstream culture lately, and is a word (or set of words) that you usually would never say while playing. Some common ones include saying your full name (with middle name) to mean stop, or using RED to mean stop and YELLOW to mean slow down, let's check in before we keep going. Don't make it something that either of you is likely to forget, and make sure that if your partner says the safeword that you stop immediately, or you may completely lose their trust.

What Do You Actually Do When You're in Charge?

You can make sexual orders, like requesting a striptease or telling them to go down on you. You could involve some impact play, which is discussed later in this section, like giving them a spanking. You could require your partner to cook or clean naked, or to give you a sensual back massage. Whatever you can dream of, you can use as part of dominating another in a sexual sense. However, it's important that you and the person submitting to you are on the same page. If you just want someone to eat you out for an hour, and your partner wants someone to pick out their clothes, order their meals, and tell them when they're allowed to orgasm, you'll want to have some good communication around compromise and what your power play interactions will actually look like.

Knowledge Gives Power

If you get more into the idea of dominating or "topping" someone, consider reading more about it. *The New Topping Book* and *The Mistress Manual* are great starter books on figuring out your dominance style and how to engage with your partner (or partners) in a way that's sexually and even emotionally fulfilling for all involved!

❥ *Sweetly Submissive*

In some of your sexiest dreams and wildest fantasies, you're kneeling at your lover's feet, with them expressing their desires and you fulfilling their every wish and command. Maybe it's incredibly freeing for you to let go and have someone else telling you what to do, or perhaps the idea of sexually serving someone to the best of your ability gets a little tingling feeling going below the belt. No matter what part of being submissive gets you going, you know that it does, and you're ready to submit.

You Still Have Power

Contrary to popular belief, being submissive or submitting to someone doesn't mean that you're weak, and it certainly doesn't mean that you're not a feminist or that you're submitting to abuse. Surprising to some people, the submissive partner is actually in charge, because during pre-play negotiations (yes, these are crucial), they set the limits on what can and cannot be done, and they also control the scene via use of their safeword. It's not abuse—kink is 100 percent consensual, and you're getting off by ALLOWING someone to be in charge of you for a designated period of time. It could be that every Saturday your partner puts a collar around your neck and you're to do anything they say that afternoon, or maybe whenever they wear black leather, you know that you're in submission to them.

Don't Go Until You Know How to Say Stop

You should always play with a safeword—this word allows you to say no without necessarily meaning it ("NO, I don't want to bend over for a spanking—make me!!"), but still allows you control of what's going on. Lots of people use RED to mean stop right now, and YELLOW to mean slow down because we need to touch base, but you could use your full name or your street address—anything that you wouldn't normally say during sexual play. Make sure you both remember it and that your partner knows that they need to stop as soon as they hear you say it.

What Do You Want?

Think for a moment or two about what makes the idea of submission so sexy to you—is it that you get to relax a little mentally and not have to be responsible for everything that's going on? Is it that calling someone Ma'am or Sir gets you wet? Are you very service oriented and just want to make your partner as happy as humanly possible?

It's important to think about WHAT you want from being submissive and communicate that to your partner. If you just have a fantasy of wanting to be "punished" for being a naughty girl by your professor who caught you, and your partner is dreaming of having a regular sex slave, you might need to touch base about each of your wants and needs, and figure out a way that everyone can get up happy. This includes discussion of how often you'll engage in power play, when you know it's time for this type of play. Do they wear a certain outfit? Do you get called a certain name? Is it a collar that you put on to indicate that you're ready to be submissive?

Power play can be just that, dominance and submission all on its own, or it can also involve other parts of kink, like bondage, or spanking, or flogging, and so on. Feel free to reach out and experiment with what works best for you.

Do Your Homework to Get in Better Trouble

If you decide that being submissive is something that you want to explore more, the *New Bottoming Book* is a great guide for someone looking into submission and "bottoming" to others. Consider reaching out to local kink groups in your area, as many have a submissives meet-up or submissives support group where you can learn more in a safe and supportive environment.

❧ *A Sexy Switch*

You don't like the idea of having to choose to be JUST a dominant sexual being or JUST a submissive sexual being. Rather, you like having options, and how you like to play with power can depend on lots of things: how you're feeling, who your partner is, and lots of other variables. You, my friend, are what the kinky community likes to call a switch—someone who can be dominant or submissive (or even something in between) depending on the situation. You might tend to be dominant with certain partners and submissive with others, or you might switch back and forth with the same partner, or even in the middle of sexual play.

Do Some Thinking Up Front

Some of your work is going to be a little more challenging than if you were "just" into domination or "just" into submission. Why? Because you have to examine both sides of your switchtastic personality and figure out what you get from partaking in each role. Is it more of a power thing, an interaction thing, a sexual thing? You need to figure out what power play looks like so that you can fulfill each set of desires. You might think that wearing a collar is really hot when you're being submissive, but you couldn't care less about collars when you're being dominant and want your partner(s) to be more specific about providing services or following certain protocol. It's going to be hard for you to share your wants and needs with current (or potential) partners if you yourself don't know what it is that gets each of those roles going for you. Do the work yourself first (potentially with the help and guidance of a friend or partner) before you start jumping back and forth and expect your lover(s) to follow along.

Communication Is Really Key

Once you've figured out what being switchy looks like to you, it's important to chat with your partner (or future partners) about how things are going to go down with power play. If your partner is only into being submissive, what might need to happen to ensure that your dominant side gets to come out and play? And if your partner is all about submission, how can you two work out some service topping or some such thing so that you get to enjoy being submissive as well? It might seem like partnering with a switch would be the best option, but then you might run into the issue of you both wanting to be more dominant at the same time. Now, that can be fun, because you could play with a sexy power struggle and whoever wins gets to bang the heck out of the other, but if one of you wants more defined roles, you need to make sure that you're able to define them before play begins.

Do Your Reading

I wish I had a go-to book to recommend, like I do for dominant folks/tops and submissive folks/bottoms, but no one has yet written *The Switching Book*. The best recommendation I can give you is the book *Playing Well with Others*, which has lots of great advice on how to, well, play well with others, predominantly in a kinky sense. There are also more and more conversations happening in kinky communities around switching—switch-focused classes, switch-focused support groups, and so on—so they could be a great resource for you in exploring what it means to be interested in power play while not feeling drawn exclusively to either a dominant or a submissive role.

Give It to Me

While there are many people who are into kink or BDSM because of the awesome power play that takes place (i.e., the whole previous section), there are also those who are attracted to kink because they like the idea of giving or receiving pain in a sexual manner. Of course, people can be into power play AND sexual pain—it doesn't have to be an either/or situation.

Usually, we call people who sexually enjoy receiving pain "masochists" and people who like giving pain in a sexual manner "sadists." However, lots of people like the idea of playing sensually with pain and don't necessarily identify with one of those terms. For example, a huge number of sexually active adults find the idea of spanking someone or being spanked to be super hot. They might not call themselves a sadist or masochist, but if hitting someone's butt (or having your own hit) gets your panties wet, this is the section for you!

There are various ways that you can "hit" someone, consensually, in a sexual way. Of these options, which one sounds the sexiest to you:

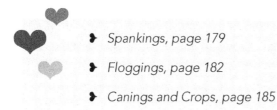

❥ *Spankings*

The concept of spanking is probably one of the most mainstream types of kink in the world. From the idea of a naughty schoolgirl getting punished over a desk to a hot pinup bending her man over her knee to give him a what for, spankings are seen as something acceptable to enjoy and therefore are frequently a starting place for people who enjoy impact play.

Make Sure Spanking Is a Happy Place

One thing to consider when you're beginning to discuss spanking with your partner: unlike other kinky things (bondage, flogging, power play), many people have experienced spanking as a "real-life" punishment when they were a child. For some people, this past experience can make the idea of spanking or being spanked that much hotter—a total reclamation of the act—but it might also be triggering for some people. It might feel a little iffy to have a conversation about it, or they might be totally gung ho when talking about it and then burst into tears the second that you begin a spanking. Just keep this in mind and make sure you're willing to help talk them through their process and are there to be supportive no matter what.

The Art of the Spank

As far as the actual spanking goes, you can use a plethora of different instruments to make the spanking happen. Of course, the cheapest and easiest to carry around with you are your hands (or your partner's hands)—you can cup them or lay them flat, and create different impact sensations, and you can have excellent control of how hard or how soft you're hitting someone.

You can begin spanking (or getting spanked) over clothes— sometimes this is a great way to start with a nice warm-up, and trust me, every good spanking has a warm-up. Just like you shouldn't go from zero to penetration in no time flat, you shouldn't go from nothing to a hardcore spanking in no time. You want to warm up the body a bit, to allow those fabulous endorphins to flow, before you start to hit too hard. Going too quickly might result in it not being fun for anyone, and usually that means that at least one party won't want to experiment with things in the future. So start out a spanking over a skirt or jeans, or at least over panties or boxers, and begin gently, even massaging the spankee in between hits. Then, once they've gotten some time to get used to the sensation, the spanker can increase the speed and intensity and really get into the spanking itself.

Spanking Supplements

Paddles are made out of all sorts of materials. Leather and wood are the most popular and look the most traditional, but paddles and slappers are now made out of silicone (great for sterilizing if you have multiple partners), corian, metal, plastic, and more. Make sure that anything that'll be hitting someone is strong and won't break. A plastic ruler might sound fun, but a cheap one might accidentally break and cut someone (wooden rulers, on the other hand, are quite sturdy and less likely to cause issues if they break). Don't want to spend the money on a fancy paddle, but want something to offset your hands? The dollar store is the place to shop; you can buy spatulas, wooden spoons, slotted pasta spoons, and much more—make an adventurous trip together to pick things out to try.

Oh, the Places You'll Spank

Where do you hit when you're spanking someone, or where should someone hit you if you're being spanked? The most popular area is obviously the buttocks, but you don't have to stop there. The back of the thighs can take a good spanking, and while it may look or feel more like slapping than spanking, you can spank/slap the inner thighs, the chest or breast area, even gently slap or spank the genitals (some people love this, some hate it—make sure you both check in with each other about whether it's pleasurable or just annoying, before you continue). The one place that you need to make sure that you don't hit at any point is the kidney area on the back—the kidneys are on either side of the spine, between the end of the rib cage and the beginning of the waist. You'll also want to be cautious around the tailbone area (between the two cheeks, sometimes called the coccyx). You should be fine when using your hands, but if you choose to use a harder or more intense implement, you'll want to make sure the spanker is aiming at one cheek or the other, rather than in between them, as one can accidentally bruise or even break the tail bone, and that would suck.

Where Is the Spank Going?

Butts can take a lot of spanking, but you'll want to check in with each other about what the goal of the spanking is. Is it a quick and gentle punishment for being naughty? Is it a way to get lots of endorphins flowing until you move to another sexual activity? Or does the person getting the spanking want to feel significant pain and have a sore butt for the next few days? All of those are completely valid options, but you want to make sure that you agree—it wouldn't be fun to put your ass in the air for a few love taps and end up barely able to sit for the next seventy-two hours, just like it might be disappointing to be craving a real beating and ending up with a few light slaps. Communication is key and will help ensure that you both enjoy your entire spanking experience.

❥ *Floggings*

When most people who have not had experience in the kink community see a flogger, they tend to call it a whip. This is a misnomer. Whips in the kink world usually are "single tails"—the type of whip that a certain Indiana Jones carried and used with skill. Be forewarned; those whips tend to be expensive and require a significant amount of practice before using them on a person. (If this is what you're interested in, I'd check out a book on single tailing, and/or join a local single tail or whips practice group.)

No, when we talk about floggers and flogging, we're referring to a solid handle with many long pieces coming off of it. They're usually made out of various types of leather, although they can be rope, Mylar, rubber, recycled tires, and many other materials.

Anatomy of a Flogger

The handle is called just that, a handle, and the long pieces coming out of it are referred to as falls. Some floggers have shorter handles, others longer, and they all have different weight. The falls can range in length from very short (a foot or less) to very long (two to three feet). Depending on the type of material (and even what animal the leather is from), the length of the falls, the width of each individual fall, whether the falls end in straight or diagonal cuts, floggers can feel either more stingy or more thuddy, and most people prefer one or the other.

Finding Your Flogger

You can get cheaply made floggers at many sex toy stores for under $50, and you can use the Internet to make one out of rope. Once you've decided that you love flogging or being flogged, you might consider investing in a good-quality flogger or two. Better-quality floggers run from around $70 to $200, depending on the material, how it's made, and so on, and need to be purchased from specialty shops or online.

Where to Flog

First, you need to know about the areas that you don't want to be hitting. Most people don't enjoy being flogged in the face (and a misplaced fall could cause some vision damage if an eye gets hit), so make sure you keep away from there. Also, the kidney area on the lower back (either side of the spine) is off-limits for impact play unless it's an incredibly gentle and almost sensual hit, so stay away from there. Keep in mind that with floggers, the falls might wrap when someone's hit, so not only does the person doing the flogging want to aim away from these areas, but they also want to think ahead and plan out where the falls might wrap, so they don't accidentally hurt someone.

Practice Makes Perfect

The best thing to do once you have a new flogger is for the person doing the flogging (yourself or your partner) to practice. Consider setting up a pillow vertically at the edge of the bed and hit it, or mark a spot on the wall to represent a person's back or front. (Yes! You can flog the chest and breast area, thighs, the tummy, etc. Just remember to stay away from the face.) Practice "throwing" the flogger (using it to hit that area), making a figure eight or infinity motions, getting into a rhythm. You can also do the occasional harder hits one or two at a time, but many people find they like being flogged in a rhythm or pace, so that they can match their breathing to it.

Advanced Technique

As the person using the flogger gets better and better, they can develop their footwork, doing the grape vine or moving back and forth as they do their flogging, rather than standing completely still. You can have two floggers of equal weights and length, and use them with one in each hand, getting into a pattern (this is frequently called Florentine). You can get different lengths and weights of floggers, and start with smaller ones and work your way up to bigger ones and vice versa. You can have the person being flogged stand with their legs slightly apart and gently flog their genitals (either naked or with underwear on) through their legs. As long as you avoid the kidney zone and the face, there's a ton of flexibility as to what you can do with a flogger.

What about the Floggee?

The person being flogged may prefer to be up against something, like a wall, so that they can brace themselves for more intense hits. If the person doing the flogging is planning to focus more on a certain area like the bottom, the receiver can bend over the edge of a bed or over a couch arm and support themselves that way. If there's a big height difference, or the person receiving cannot stand for long, you can have them straddle a chair backward so that their back remains available, but they're also supported in various ways throughout the flogging.

Cold, Warm, Warmer, Hot!

Like spankings, canings, and really, all sexual acts, you want to warm up the person being flogged, rather than just hitting them super hard from square one. This approach allows their skin to warm up, to get used to being hit by something (especially since this usually doesn't happen regularly), and gets those wonderfully useful endorphins coursing through the body.

Keep Communication Up

Check in, especially when you first start flogging, to see if both of you are on the same page about how hard the hits are. In fact, the person doing the flogging should have the other partner hit them a few times with the flogger first to give them an idea of how hard it lands and how it feels, so they can know what type of sensation they're giving. And although a flogging might leave less intense bruises than a hardcore over-the-knee spanking or a more intense caning, flogging can definitely end up leaving some marks, so make sure you discuss if that's OK—and where it's acceptable to have those marks—before you get started.

❥ *Canings and Crops*

You're interested in something a little more off the road than your run-of-the-mill spanking, and you're not sure if the whole flogger thing is right for you. Luckily, you can be kinky and provide (or receive) some awesome impact play using canes or crops (or both!). Frequently, when you hear the word *cane*, you might think of a walking stick or cane used for support during walking. While those certainly COULD be used to hit someone, most people who like giving and receiving canings prefer to do so with thinner canes made of rattan, bamboo, acrylic, or fiberglass. As far as crops, yes, they're exactly like those things they use to make horses go faster, except that in this case, they're designed to make a human get lots of endorphins exploding faster and turn some of that pain into pleasure.

Let's Talk Canes

You could absolutely go to your local open space or forest (though not a national park—that's illegal) and pick yourself a birch or willow cane for use on yourself or your partner. In the real world, many kink folks prefer to have premade canes specifically designed for use on humans, have no risk of splinters or random bugs, and have convenient handles attached, making them more comfortable to use than a small branch you picked out of the woods.

The rule of thumb on canes is that the thinner and more flexible it is, the more sting there will be in the hit. The wider and more rigid it is, the thuddier and deeper the hit will be. Some people like the look and feel of wood, and you can get rattan and bamboo canes for a pretty low price of $10–$20 and up, depending on the quality of the wood, the type of handle, and so on. Acrylic canes provide a slightly different sensation and are usually very flexible (read: very stingy), while fiberglass canes are more rigid, providing a more thuddy and harder hit. You can find canes at specialty kink stores both online and in the real world, and sometimes you can find them in other places and repurpose them for sexual use.

Canes Leave Marks

Period. Yes, there may be those few special people out there who don't particularly bruise from a good caning, but for the most part, canes are going to leave long-line bruises wherever they hit. These marks can take a day or two to show up (so you can't really go on whether someone is bruised by the time you're finished playing together). If the person who likes impact play on the receiving end can't have any bruises, caning is not for you at this point. On the other hand, some people love the bruises they get and even enjoy making patterns out of the cane marks (a tic-tac-toe board, anyone?).

Where Caning Feels Best

The best places to cane someone are on the buttocks and the thighs (front, back, and even the inner regions), and even the bottoms of the feet, although those REALLY hurt when hit. You definitely want to stay away from anywhere the bone is closer to the skin, like shins, forearms, spinal area, and so on, as well as avoiding the face and the neck.

Canes Are Serious(ly Fun)

Keep in mind that caning is more intense than flogging or spanking. There are less creative things you can do with canes, but they serve their purpose well. Make sure that whoever is giving the caning starts slow and provides a nice, long warm-up to get the receiver's body ready for the more intense sensations, and gives the body enough time to start producing some incredibly awesome endorphins that help make everything feel even better and more sexual.

All about Crops

As far as crops, they also sting, but in a much more specific and directed area than a cane, because the tip of a crop is only a few inches long at most and an inch or two wide. Of course, there are traditional crops, designed for use on horses (available at your local equestrian supply store, as well as at specialty kink shop storefronts and online), but there are more fun and entertaining crops on the market, like a skull crop, a rose crop, a star crop, a kitty crop, and more. Most crops are made of leather, but there is also the Lollicrop (yes, a crop that looks like a lollipop), where the crop's tip is made of silicone, providing for some unique and different sensations from the more frequently used leather crops.

Just Like with a Horse, Crops Can Direct

Crops are great because while you certainly can use them separately for impact play, they're also easy to integrate into other types of sexual play. For example, if your partner is going down on you, you could use the crop to give them directions and speed instructions, just like a jockey gives a horse. A hit on their left shoulder can mean more to the left, right shoulder more to the right, and hitting their back can determine the speed. You can also use crops to hit genitals, since crops have nice compact tips that make aiming easier. Keep in mind that warm-ups are important with all types of impact play, so start with gentle hits that are fewer and farther between, and work yourself up to more intense and quicker hits once the receiver has gotten their bearings.

Bound by Love

In the previous section, I debunked the idea behind whips (what most people think are whips are in actuality floggers), and for this section, it's time to debunk the concept behind chains. While some people may wind up using chains, most people who enjoy indulging in bondage never actually consider chains. They're cold, bulky, heavy, noisy, and hard to use. In the real world, people usually use something they have lying around such as a scarf or tie, or they invest in good quality cuffs, or they learn some tips and techniques of rope play.

Caution: Frequently, people interested in experimenting with bondage either pick up cheap novelty handcuffs (including those covered with fake fur or marabou feathers) or get themselves a pair of more heavy-duty handcuffs. While these are fun ideas as props for a hot cop role-play, I strongly advise against using them for actual bondage where someone might be pulling against them. The metal, even the cheap aluminum in the novelty cuffs, can cut into the skin and possibly cause nerve damage. Instead, keep reading for some other fun and fabulous options for bondage that are safer for everyone involved.

If you're interested in exploring bondage (you love the idea of being tied up or tying someone up), which of the following most interests you?

❥ *Silky Scarves and Tantalizing Neck Ties, page 189*

❥ *Captivating Cuffs, page 191*

❥ *Rocking Ropes, page 194*

❥ *Silky Scarves and Tantalizing Neck Ties*

You're raring to go with this whole bondage thing, but you'd rather use what you have around the house than invest in some leather cuffs or spend hours memorizing rope ties. For you, that sensuous and soft scarf would be perfect for tying up your lover, or that necktie that your partner always wears would look absolutely lovely around your ankles. Maybe you enjoy the perversion of normal everyday things being used sexually, or maybe you just don't want to have to think about where to get and then store special bondage items—either way, household goods are perfect for you.

The Perfect Pick

Scarves and ties can make great and comfortable items to create bondage. Just keep in mind that when you decide to use things like these to tie up someone or get tied up, you probably shouldn't use your absolutely favorite tie or expensive scarf. Why not? Because fabric, of all kinds, tends to tighten its knots when anything pulls against it. This means that if one of you is tied up and experiencing sexual pleasure, resulting in you pulling against your bonds, the knot in the fabric may tighten so much that you need to cut it to get it off. This means that (1) you should have a pair of EMT or safety shears on hand (they have dull tips, so no skin gets cut if you have to cut things off of the body), and (2) you don't want to use an item that would leave you heartbroken if ruined.

On a side note, this is why using nylons or pantyhose for bondage is a really bad idea—their super-stretchy material pulls very tight VERY fast, and in addition to making it impossible to get the knots undone, this also means that the knots can tighten too much and actually cut off circulation, which is never a good thing to have happen.

Know Your Knots

One easy way to solve the issue of knots becoming too tight is to make a slipknot out of the scarf or tie, slip it around the wrist or ankle of the person being restrained, and then tie it to the edge of the bed, a leg of a chair, and so on. That means you can tie a bow that's easy to remove when tying it to the actual tie point, and the slipknot will allow you to loosen the ties should you need to in the middle of playing. Keep in mind that if you want to be sexually active with someone once they're tied up, you should probably think about the position they're tied in. Are their legs open? Are their genitals accessible? Is it a comfortable position for both of you to engage in various sexual activities?

Time and Place

Double looping the tie or scarf around the body parts you're tying helps distribute the pressure so that your partner can be comfortably tied for a longer time. The person tied up should let their partner know if they start losing sensation in their hands or feet, and the person not tied up should check to make sure limbs don't get really cold or turn colors, which indicates circulation problems. Especially in the beginning, don't tie each other up for too long. You can always take a break to get the blood flowing and then get tied up in a new position. Also, make sure that the ties are not exactly ON a wrist or ankle joint; place them just above or below the joint. This is a safety precaution, to ensure that you're putting pressure not directly on the joint but instead, on the surrounding muscle.

❥ *Captivating Cuffs*

When it comes to bondage, you like things that are easy, look good, and are safe. Getting a pair or two of good cuffs is going to make bondage that much easier and that much more awesome for you and your partner. Cuffs are easy on and easy off, making quick work of getting tied up or tying someone up, and when playtime is over, they're super simple to take off and toss aside. There are no fancy tricks to learn, and cuffs never get pulled too tight, so you don't have to ever worry about cutting them off. Cuffs are cool like that.

Know Your Cuffs

While most wrist and ankle cuffs are made of leather, they also can be made of metal (like steel shackles), nylon webbing, faux fur, vinyl, and more. Be VERY careful using metal: when you pull tight against it, you can suffer serious nerve damage. Cheap cuffs are available at almost every run-of-the-mill sex shop or adult store, or you can invest in a higher-quality and longer-lasting set from a specialty kink shop or online. Some cuffs come with fur on the inside for added comfort—many folks like how that feels, although others might find that their sex play gets too hot and sweaty for fur to be pressed up against anyone's body.

If you're just starting out, a cheap nylon or fake leather set will work just fine, but if bondage becomes something that you do regularly, you may want to invest in a nice pair that's more comfortable, less likely to break, and will last for years to come. Smaller cuffs are great for wrists, while larger ones are for ankles. If you or your partner has extra large wrists, consider getting ankle cuffs for use on the wrists, and if someone's ankles are tiny, you can always use wrist cuffs if they fit.

Cuff Stuff

Once someone is cuffed, then what? How do you use these things? There are many options! You can loop the D rings together and just hold them in your hand, especially if the bondage is more for show than inhibiting motion. You can use rope (or scarves) to tie the D rings together, or use rope to tie the cuffs to the bed, around a chair, and so on. You can invest in a few cheap snap hooks or carabiners from your local home improvement store and use those to hook the cuffs together or to anchor points.

How do you make anchor points? If you're super serious about using bondage in your sex life, you can always sink eyelets and hooks into your walls (maybe check with your landlord first if you're a renter), but just remember that your average eyelet in the wall should not be used to bear weight. If you don't want to do any kind of permanent damage to the walls, you might consider investing in the Sportsheets Under the Bed Restraint system. It's a brilliant design—it has nylon webbing straps in kind of an X shape. You put the middle of the X between your mattress and box spring, and then each leg of the X hangs out at the corners of your bed. At the end of each X leg is a D ring and a snap hook, so you can either hook or tie each of your cuffs to them, putting someone in a spread-eagle position. The person's weight on the bed, as well as the X design (if you pull one side, it pulls on the limb that's on the other side), makes everything stay in place. When you're done playing, you just tuck the legs of the X under the bed and no one will ever see them. The system comes with velour Velcro cuffs, but you can absolutely use your own cuffs instead.

Just for Show, or More to Know

If you like the look of leather and a collar, you might even choose to wear restraints as part of your power play situation, even if you don't use them for bondage. You can also hook ankle cuff to wrist cuff, or hook both wrist cuffs to someone's collar, or even flip someone on their stomach and hook their cuffs into a basic hogtie. While cuffs will not get tighter or loose when pulled on (like scarves and even rope sometimes), the person who's not wearing them should definitely check on the person who is, to see if their hands and feet are getting cold and are turning colors, both of which indicate lack of circulation. Cuffs are nice because you can loosen or tighten them during play, so that if someone starts slipping out, you can tighten them, or you can restore circulation during play simply by loosening the cuffs instead of having to cut someone loose and start again.

❥ *Rocking Ropes*

The idea of using rope to create beautiful bondage situations really turns you on. Perhaps the feeling of the rope against your skin as you're bound or in your fingers as you tie up your partner makes your breath catch, or maybe you've seen some gorgeous rope ties and like the look of them. Whatever the case may be, rope gets you going, and that's the medium that you'd like to use as you explore the brilliance of bondage.

Ancient Art or Improv

There are a few camps of rope folks out there. Some practice Shibari, which is a centuries-old Japanese practice of rope tying. Others focus on different historical and cultural styles of doing rope. Still others just tie people however they feel at that moment and don't follow any particular style or custom. However YOU feel that you want to learn to tie rope is the right way for you, so don't let anyone who likes a particular style or way of doing rope tell you that other ways are wrong or bad. That being said, there are a few things you need to keep in mind for safety when using rope.

Safety First—Seriously

First and foremost, if you're tying up anyone with rope or being tied up, make sure you have a pair of EMT shears or safety scissors on hand. These are super-sharp scissors with blunt tips—they can cut through pennies, but if you have to slide them under a rope to cut it off, the blunt tips prevent skin cuts. Sure, you might say that you're not doing anything serious or complicated with rope, but I don't care, get some shears anyway. What would happen if your partner or you were tied up and then the fire alarm went off, or your mother-in-law stopped by for a surprise visit? Knots that might be easily undone in calm situations can be absolutely impossible to budge under pressure. Better to be safe than sorry: get the shears.

Next, make sure that you think about where you're putting rope. It should never go around your partner's neck or your neck, not even for play. Again, think about the worst-case scenario: if one of you passed out and your body put pressure on the rope, you definitely wouldn't want it to cut off the windpipe. Just don't do it. To tie joints, put the rope slightly below or slightly above ankles, wrists, knees, and elbows, rather than directly on the joint—this removes pressure from the joint, so that the person tied up won't risk injuring their joint if they pull. Also, you should wrap rope at least two times around each area being tied—the more wraps, the less pressure on the area, and the more comfortable it is.

Rope Shopping
The type of rope that you buy depends on how serious you are about learning to do rope and what you're going to use it for. Total beginners can buy cheap cotton clothesline or cotton rope by the foot at the local hardware store. If you want a specific color, many sex toy and specialty kink stores sell black, pink, purple, naturally colored, and other colors of rope in different lengths. If you're really getting into using rope, you can look for different materials like hemp, jute, coconut, and more. Again, it's all about what you want from it—if you're just starting out and aren't sure if you and your partner are going to like using rope, buy something cheap and easy to begin with and upgrade once you decide that you love using rope.

Knot Homework
If you're brand-new to rope, you might consider picking up a kinky rope book that's full of information on different types of ties that

you can use. *Shibari You Can Use: Japanese Rope Bondage and Erotic Macramé, The Seductive Art of Japanese Rope Bondage, Bondage for Sex,* and *Two Knotty Boys Showing You the Ropes: A Step-by-Step, Illustrated Guide for Tying Sensual and Decorative Rope Bondage* are all awesome step-by-step guides that teach you different types of rope work that you can practice on your partner or have your partner practice on you (or you can even take turns, switching it up, so that you both learn). In addition to using rope for bondage, you can also learn how to make decorative body harnesses, rope gauntlets, and more. Once you get good, you can even learn some tricks about putting a knot right on the clit or testicles, so that if whoever is tied up wiggles a bit, they get an extra nice surprise.

Chapter

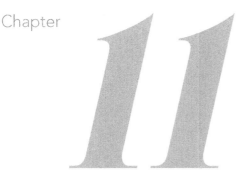

Safer Is Sexy — How to Protect Yourself and Your Partner

For most people, having a chat about sexually transmitted infections and sexual histories isn't the most fun thing they ever do. In fact, most people are so scared, nervous, or just not into talking about these things that they choose not to have these conversations, which is unfortunate. And if you haven't had this talk, deciding on which form of protection to use can be given short shrift.

First, we need to recognize that there's no such thing as 100 percent safe sex, unless you're masturbating and getting yourself off in the ways that you like best. The second you bring someone else (or someONES, who knows!) into the sexual equation, there's a hint of risk that exists. Even kissing someone puts you at risk for getting the common cold or cold sores (which most people don't realize is one strain of the herpes simplex virus). Now, this doesn't mean that you should never be sexually active, but it does mean that you need to be thoughtful about your sexual interactions so that you can have the information needed to protect yourself in whichever ways you deem necessary.

In this chapter, I talk about the following:

X--- How to have the safer-sex talk by being front and center, dipping a toe in, or beating around the bush.

X--- What safer sex looks like when it comes to toys, oral, and handiwork.

How to Have the Safer-Sex Talk

Something that's crucial to talk about not only for safer sex but also for sexually transmitted infections is that there's nothing wrong with having an STI. In fact, 80 percent of sexually active American woman currently have, or have had, a sexually transmitted infection at some point in their lives. About 75 percent of sexually active folks have the human papillomavirus (commonly called HPV), and while there are a few strains that cause cervical cancer and one that causes genital warts, there are a total of 110 strains of HPV.

Many people with an STI don't even know that they have it. A lot of folks, particularly men, tend not to show symptoms of having an STI and so are carriers without even realizing it. Plus, lots of people don't get STI tests regularly, and many doctors don't do full-panel testing (again, especially not on men), so a lot of people aren't aware of their STI status with any accuracy.

What Does This Mean?

It means that we need to turn this conversation about "clean" and "not clean" on its head. Saying that you're clean because you don't have an STI is ridiculous. First of all, you might not even know for sure whether you're positive or negative for all the STIs that exist in the world, and second, cleanliness has nothing to do with whether or not you're positive. Being clean means that you shower or bathe regularly and practice good hygiene. Being negative means that you've had a recent FULL-panel of STI tests, and they all came back negative.

Now that we've got that out of the way, let's talk safer sex conversations. They're usually not going to be super exciting, but they don't have to be boring or uncomfortable. Depending on how you best communicate, as well as the situation that you're in (a hookup in a bar bathroom might be a very different conversation from one with a long-term, monogamous partner), you can figure out how to have these talks in a way that's helpful and satisfactory for all involved.

When you begin to have the safer sex conversation, you'll need to decide which communication style is best for you. Of the following options, which one resonates best:

❥ *Front and Center, page 200*

❥ *Dipping in a Toe, page 201*

❥ *Beating around the Bush, page 203*

❥ *Front and Center*

You want to be crystal clear and to the point, no sugarcoating of anything. Good for you. If everyone could be this direct in conversations about sex and sexuality, the world would be a very different place. It's important to remember that not everyone feels that way about conversations on sexuality, so you can go in being no-nonsense, but know that you might need to practice a little patience and diplomacy for people who aren't yet ready to be this open.

Just the Facts, Ma'am

Before you get started, you need to get your ducks in a row. When was the last time you were STI tested? What were you tested for? Many people know their HIV, herpes, gonorrhea, and chlamydia statuses, but have no idea where they stand about HPV, trichomoniasis, or syphilis or even whether they were at risk for hepatitis C. Know which STIs you've been tested for and what the results were. You can be a carrier for herpes without ever having had an outbreak, so make sure that you've had a blood test if you're going to tell people that you're herpes negative.

Next, think about what the ideal safer sex situation is for you. What needs to be covered, when does it need to be covered, and who's responsible for providing the protection? What activities are OK without protection (if any) and what activities require protection (if any)?

Time to Talk

Now that you have a fairly decent base of where you are, go for the talk. Make sure that you let your partner know what you're doing and the topic, so you aren't going from a hot and heavy make-out session directly into a serious STI discussion without some sort of transition. Lay your cards on the table with the information above, and ask them for their info—date of last testing, what they were tested for, and their statuses. Talk about what activities you might be interested in doing, and what safer sex looks like for each of them. Discuss who's bringing the safer sex supplies, who decides when they go on, and so on.

Talk Fast

Of course, if this is a quickie in the bar bathroom, you could sidle up to your newest amour and just show them your gloves/condoms/dam and say, "Let's go for it—sound good?" Not every safer sex conversation needs to be a long-term negotiation. If you're ready to get it on, go for it and have fun, making sure that you always go with the highest common denominator of safer sex. If only one of you cares about protection for intercourse, and the other one wants it for intercourse AND oral sex, the highest common denominator is using protection for intercourse AND oral sex, so that's what you should do.

❥ *Dipping in a Toe*

You're ready to have the conversation. You know it's important, and you want to make yourself as safe as possible during your sexual journey. You know all of this, yet you're not quite ready to put it all out there in an open conversation. That's just fine.

Break the Ice

Start by feeling things out. You can ask when someone last had their annual physical, and ask whether they had any STI testing done then. You could talk about "your friend" and how she and her partner just had the tricky safer sex conversation, and you wonder how it might go with the two of you. You can bring up the flavored condoms or dam that you saw at the drugstore, and ask your partner what type of safer sex protections they prefer to use. There are many ways to ease into this conversation.

Take the Test Together

You might find that one of you, or maybe even both of you, have not had STI testing done recently. If you're looking at a short-term or long-term relationship (as compared with a one-night stand), you might consider making a date out of it. You can both schedule your testing at a doctor's office, clinic, or Planned Parenthood, and go in together (they'll probably have you tested in two different rooms, because they prefer to ask some screening questions one-on-one, but you can wait in the lobby together). After getting tested, go out and get some ice cream or cupcakes, and celebrate being on top of your sexual health. You'll both get your results at the same time in a few weeks and can celebrate again by knowing your statuses, deciding what safer sex barriers you want to use, and doing the deed to seal the deal.

For a Shortie

If you're in a short-term one-night or one-weekend (or one-vacation) stand, then getting tested together is not an option. You could both write down what safer sex means, and switch papers, or have a moderately candid discussion while watching TV or driving somewhere. If you're not sure that you're ready to have an in-depth talk about the last time you were each tested, you can always just forgo the conversation in favor of a visual—show them the condoms, gloves, and dams you have ready to go, and say, "We'll be using these to protect each other … any questions?" Problem solved.

❥ *Beating around the Bush*

Perhaps you're new to the whole safer sex conversation because you just got out of a long-term monogamous relationship that didn't use any type of barriers, or you could just be shy when it comes to discussing what's happening below the belt. That's absolutely fine, but it doesn't let you off the hook for figuring out how to have a conversation with your current partner (or partners) about safer sex and how to practice it as part of your sexual interactions.

Slow and Steady

Begin slow, and begin with yourself. Think about the last time that you had an STI test. If it wasn't within the last six months to a year, then it's probably time that you took care of that, at the very least for your own peace of mind. Most insurance plans cover STI testing as part of your wellness exam. Feel free to ask your doctor what is and isn't covered, and to ask for a full panel. If you don't have insurance, or for some reason they don't cover your testing, lots of clinics and Planned Parenthoods offer reduced price or sliding scale options on getting tested for sexually transmitted infections. Additionally, if you live in a big city or a county affected by high STI rates, many organizations and health departments will offer free testing for HIV and other STIs, and they may also offer free treatment and vaccinations.

Prep Your Speech

Once you have some good information for yourself on your statuses and where you stand, you can think about what safer sex looks like to you. Do you want to be in charge of bringing the supplies (condoms, gloves, dams, etc.), or do you want your partner in charge of that? Maybe you could take turns? What activities are a must for safer sex, and which ones don't matter to you about whether or not you practice safer sex (some people couldn't care less about using gloves for manual stimulation/hand jobs/handiwork, while for others, it's an absolute requirement!)? Who's responsible for getting out the barriers and using them? You need to have this figured out in your mind before you share it with your partner.

If you think you might be ready to sit down and talk, consider scheduling a time for it, so you both are able to prepare. It's absolutely OK at the beginning of a talk to share that you don't feel super comfortable having this conversation, but that you care very much about the state of your own sexual health, as well as that of your partner. They may feel the same way, and you can move forward awkwardly together. If they're comfortable with the conversation, letting them know that you might be a little more hesitant can give them the signal to slow down a little and think about how they discuss these things.

A Virtual Talk

Are you super anxious and not ready to have this talk face-to-face? Maybe you're not ready to be sexually active with someone whom you can't talk to about safer sex. But if you're bashful about talking and totally sure of wanting to get it on, you can always have the conversation via IM, text message, or e-mail. Remember, it's an incredibly important conversation to have, even if you're feeling nervous about it. Your own sexual health is crucial, and this will help you feel confident in protecting yourself now and in future situations. Consider practicing in front of a mirror, with a friend, or by writing out your thoughts.

Most of all, never back down. If you need a certain level of protection for a certain activity to make you feel comfortable in protecting your body, don't let anyone convince you otherwise. Safer sex and decisions about your own sexual health are choices that YOU make, and they're not silly or high maintenance, and don't have anything to do with whether you love or trust someone. You get to make the decisions for your body. Period.

What Safer Sex Looks Like

OK, so you've had the conversation about safer sex and what that looks like to the two of you. Mazel tov! Great, but the conversation doesn't end there. You need to know how to practice safer sex. If you're like lots of people out there, you didn't get an accurate and inclusive look at safer sex and what barriers to use during different types of sex. Don't worry! We're going to cover it right here and right now.

When you're thinking about safer sex, think about each activity and what type of safer sex supplies you might need for each. Which activity below might you want to learn more about regarding safer sex?

- *Insertables: Toys and Penises, page 206*
- *Oral Action: Cunnilingus, Fellatio, and Analingus, page 210*
- *Delightful Digits: Handiwork of All Sorts, page 212*

❧ *Insertables: Toys and Penises*

Lots of people like to put things in their bodies, and frequently those things are dildos, plugs, other toys, and penises. The easiest way to have safer sex with most of these things is to use condoms.

The Classic Condom

Condoms were originally made out of cloth bags with drawstrings. I'm sure you don't have to be a super-scientific person to know that they weren't quite as useful as modern condoms. While perhaps they lowered the rate of pregnancy, they weren't exactly dependable in preventing pregnancy. Given this, people started using "lambskin" for condoms, which is a nice way of saying sheep intestines. While you can still get lambskin condoms today, both the originals and the modern version aren't capable of preventing the transmission of sexually transmitted infections (although they're much more adept at preventing pregnancy than cloth bags). So if you're in the market for something that prevents the transmission of STIs, you need a condom made of latex or one of the non-latex options such as polyurethane or polyisoprene condoms.

Condoms All the Way

For vaginal and anal intercourse with a penis, a condom is the ONLY way to practice safer sex that prevents or reduces the transmission of sexually transmitted infections, period. There's nothing that you can eat, douche with, spray on, and so on that will work. Condoms are the end-all, be-all.

Nowadays you have the option of "male" condoms (you know, the ones that you see all the time, in the small 1" by 1" square packages, that roll down on a penis or sex toy) or "female" condoms that have two rings in them and are a bit looser (and are all latex-free).

Handling a Condom Correctly

To use a "male" condom on a penis, first check the expiration date and make sure it's still good. Then feel the package to make sure that there's some air inside. Gently tear it open along the edge (as sexy as it may sound to use your teeth to tear it open, that's a great way to accidentally tear the condom, rendering it useless). Now, hold it up and look at which way it rolls down. Note: If you put it on upside down, you absolutely CANNOT just flip it. Pre-cum or pre-ejaculate can contain both semen and STIs — if you flip it, you'll be putting that directly into your body. If this happens, you need to toss out that condom and start again.

Once you have it the right direction, put a drop or two of non-water-based lube either inside the tip of the condom or on the tip of the penis — having the lube between the condom and the penis will increase sensation for the wearer (you don't need a ton of lube here — just a drop or two will suffice). Pinch the tip lightly, and roll the condom down onto the base of the penis.

Now, do whatever you want, although remember to keep anything with oil in it away from latex condoms (massage oil, lotion, chocolate sauce, etc.). Once you're finished, move the penis away from the mouth, vulva, or anus, and carefully remove the condom — taking care not to spill anything — and tie a knot in the end. Wrap it in tissue or toilet paper, and throw it in the trash. DO NOT flush condoms — they can break your septic or sewer system. If you have kids or pets, you may want to ensure it's in a closeable trash can, or take the trash out to prevent them from finding it.

Condoms on the Loose

Sometimes people ask about losing a condom—if you put a condom IN someone (mouth, vagina, or anus), you should make sure that you have said condom when you're done. If for some reason it comes off, you should reach in and remove it. Don't let a condom stay inside someone after sex; it can cause infections. If you lose it in the anus and can't get it out, you must go to the doctor and have it removed. If you or your partner is having trouble getting the condom to stay on, hold the base of it during sex or use a cock ring to help hold it in place.

Female Form

To use a "female" condom with a penis, check the package's expiration date first to ensure that it's still good, and make sure that the package isn't ripped or torn. Carefully open it up and find the two rings (internal and external). Then, lubricate the vulva or anus, squeeze the internal ring, and slip it into the body, taking care that the external ring stays outside the body. Insert penis, and have fun (you may want one of you to hold the external ring in place to make sure it doesn't slip or get accidentally pushed into the body). When you're done, remove the condom, wrap it up in either tissue or toilet paper, and put it in the trash. Don't even think about flushing it—you'd back up your toilet faster than you can say "barrier method." If you have kids or pets, figure out a way to keep it away from them.

Wrapping Up Sex Toys

What about with sex toys? Sex toys can absolutely transmit STIs from person to person, and if not properly cleaned or protected, they can actually give someone back a UTI or yeast infection that they had before.

Some sex toy materials can be sterilized. If your dildo, butt plug, or what have you is 100 percent medical grade silicone, glass, ceramic, or metal, you can boil it for three to five minutes, wash it on the top shelf of the dishwasher, or wipe it down with a 10 percent bleach solution (let it dry and then wash it off). Doing so will completely sterilize the toy, making it safer to use with a new partner or with yourself if you're worried about retransmitting something to yourself.

If you own a sex toy that's not sterilizable (anything not listed above), or you don't have the time, energy, or wherewithal to sterilize it before you use it with someone, you're going to want to condom it up. You can have the person being penetrated use a "female" condom as listed above for anal or vaginal penetration, or you can slip a "male" condom on the toy. You don't need to worry about putting lube inside the condom, since sensation of the toy is a nonissue. However, you definitely want to wrap the used condom in tissue or toilet paper and throw it away after play is over (do NOT flush it—it'll clog up your system). You should wash your toy if you're using a lubricated or powdered condom, just to keep it clean—soap and warm water will do the trick. You can also use condoms over vibrators for external use and over butt plugs and other anal toys. Anything that touches genital areas is at risk for the transmission of STIs. Better to be safe than sorry.

Note on insertables: If you're going from the vagina to the anus, you don't need to change condoms, and ditto from mouth to vagina, and vagina to mouth. On the other hand, if you're going from anus to vagina or anus to mouth, you 100 percent absolutely need to change condoms or risk giving the receiver all sorts of not fun bacterial infections.

❥ *Oral Action: Cunnilingus, Fellatio, and Analingus*

For cunnilingus (oral-vulvar) and analingus (oral-anal), you can use a dam or make your own dam out of a glove, condom, or cling wrap. Now that I've said that, you're probably wondering, what's a dam?

Dam Good Invention

While the condom has been around for literally centuries, until the 1970s and 1980s people giving and receiving analingus and cunnilingus had no way to protect themselves and their partners during oral sex. They started out by using the dams that dentists used during cavity fillings, which were big, blue, and thick. They didn't allow for transmission of any STIs, which was great, but they also didn't allow for much transmission of any sensation either, which was less than fabulous. They reached out to condom companies and asked them to create latex dams made out of material that was thinner and more similar to condoms.

Modern dams are very thin sheets of latex (similar in feeling to a condom) that are rectangular and usually flavored—purple is grape, green is mint, and so on. All you have to do is lube up the area that's going to be licked, place the dam on top of it, and go for the gold! The problems with dams are that they tend to be hard to find, so you'll likely need to order them online or get them at a sex positive toy store; they're expensive ($2–$3 PER dam!); and they aren't great for those with latex sensitivities. Good news—there are options!

DIY Safer Sex Supplies

Hooray! Now it's time to MacGyver your safer sex supplies! There are a few ways to make dams of your own on the cheap, and also in latex-free options. One way is to take an unrolled condom and cut it in half, from tip to the base (lengthwise). Voilà—you have a mini dam, and you can even use flavored condoms, lubricated or not, or non-latex condoms. You can find flavored condoms at most supermarkets, drugstores, and sex toy/adult shops. Keep in mind that some flavored lubricants may contain glycerin, so check on that if either you or your partner happens to be sensitive to glycerin. Definitely do NOT use spermicidal condoms for oral action, as they tend to taste nasty and cause irritation or allergic reactions in a lot of people.

Another great trick for dam creation is to take a glove (latex, nitrile, or vinyl—your choice!), cut off the four finger spaces, and up along the edge on the NON-thumb side. Open it up, and now you have a dam with a little finger hole for you to stimulate inside as well. Gloves are cheap in bulk, and you can find them at supermarkets, drugstores, or even beauty supply shops. Plus, they come in lots of color options, which can be fun—you can match them to your lingerie, bedroom walls, or even car interior (whatever works for you!). Just remember that if you or your partner has a latex allergy, stick with either the nitrile or the vinyl options.

Once last super-easy way to make an alternative dam is to use cling wrap or plastic wrap from the kitchen. The nice thing is that most people already have this on hand, it comes in pretty colors, and you can see what's beneath the wrap so you can enjoy what you're licking. Plus, all plastic wrap is latex-free, so it works even if one or both of you have a latex allergy. Heck, you could even build an ice cream sundae on top of the cling wrap, because it wouldn't be near the vulva or anus, and you could really enjoy yourself as you ate someone out (or vice versa, of course!).

Lend a Hand

During oral sex, you can even have the person receiving oral sex hold the dam or barrier to help out and feel more involved. Does that sound like it's still going to be too much work for you or your partner? Good news! There are fancy dam-holder harnesses (so not kidding). If that's too out in left field or cost prohibitive, the receiver of oral sex can wear a garter belt and use the straps or clips to hold the barrier in place, making for hands-free oral action. Plus, if the dam or barrier is pulled tightly, it transmits humming VERY well, and that can feel amazing for the person getting the oral action.

Lube Is AMAZING

People frequently complain that dams and condoms during oral sex "ruin the sensation." Never fear—there's a trick! Use some good lubricant between the barrier and the genitals (anus, vulva, or penis) to help transmit the sensations being provided. Think of it as a safer sex sandwich—genitals, lube, barrier, tongue and mouth. You can read more about lubes in the lubricants section.

❥ *Delightful Digits: Handiwork of All Sorts*

Are you someone who loves some nice fingering, hand jobs, or other handiwork action? Bring on the gloves! Gloves to use for sex are easy to find—most supermarkets and drugstores have them (look for medical or beauty gloves), but if you want fun colors, look online for gloves marketed to tattoo artists and doctor's offices. You can find them in almost every color of the rainbow, and even in black. Sexy, right? Some people think that gloves are hot. You can make them part of a latex outfit, or help with some medical role-play. Things to think about!

The Benefits of Glove Love

Why might you want to wear gloves during sex? Not only can STIs be transmitted person to person via vaginal fluid or semen on hands, but gloves are truly amazing and useful for many reasons. If the person doing the fingering/manual stimulating/hand jobbing has hang nails or long nails or sharp nails, using gloves can help prevent the person being pleasured from getting small cuts and tears in and around their vagina, anus, or penis. Plus, if we're talking vaginal fingering, vaginal fluid tends to be slightly acidic, so if you're spending time playing around there, gloves can protect hands from feeling a slight stinging in small cuts and rough patches. If the person giving the pleasure has long nails, you can pop half a cotton ball into the tip of each finger in the glove before putting it on, and they're no longer a hazard for their partner's genitals. Also, some people have jobs that rough up their hands, or they might work with corrosive chemicals — this can really hurt the delicate skin on and around the genitals. Using gloves can help make this a nonissue.

Not only that, but gloves can help any lubricant you're using (both natural and store bought) last longer. Since humans are water based and are about 80 percent water, our bodies tend to absorb water-based lubrication (including the type that bodies produce) much faster than a gloved surface does.

One last bonus of wearing gloves is that they can make for much quicker clean up, or moving to the next sexual activity, or cuddling. No need to get up, wash hands with soap and water, dry them off, and head back in for more action.

Chapter

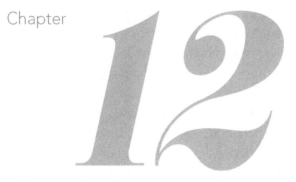

Where to Go from Here?

Here we are. You've followed *Your Pleasure Map* down all its treasure trails. If you picked your way through the book, I hope that you found what you were looking for or even stumbled on something that you didn't even know you were looking for. If not, consider going back through and choosing some of the choices that you skipped over and seeing what else there is to learn.

The concept of a map is one that works well for sex. There are lots of locations, and each area has many paths and ways of getting there. Sure, you may want to take the well-traveled highways that you know to be safe and easy. But you also might meander along the side roads, taking longer to get to your destination but truly enjoying your journey. Of course, you might be one of those trailblazers who prefers to follow your own path, or even travel how the bird flies. Sex, sexuality, and relationships are like that—there are different activities that may lead to various end points, but there's no magically correct or "right" way to get there.

I hope that you learned at least one new thing in reading this book. That's always my goal for everyone who comes to one of my classes or reads my books: to learn one thing that's completely new and different. Maybe it was the length of the clitoris or something about anal play. Perhaps it was the hint of something new about playing with power or tricks and techniques of safer sex that you had never thought of before. I ask that you take that new thing and share it far and wide among friends, coworkers, your coffee klatch, weight-lifting group, or knitting circle.

Women deserve more information, particularly more accurate information about how to feel empowered sexually. We no longer live in the Victorian world of hush-hush conversations and avoidance of the word *clitoris*. Rather, we should all be able to have good conversations about sexual pleasure, satisfaction, and more while feeling confident in asking for our needs and wants to be met by our partners. Conversely, we should feel good in pleasing our partners, not because we feel that we have to or because we believe that sex is some tit-for-tat type of thing, but because we like doing it and we know that we're good at it. Every woman, well, truly, every adult, should be able to have whatever knowledge they crave about sex, anatomy, relationships, communication, and more without ever feeling an ounce of guilt or shame about being sexually educated and empowered.

This book is not the end-all and be-all of sexuality information. I encourage you to keep being hungry for knowledge. Read a book that's all about anal or delves into pegging. Watch an educational porn on threesomes or oral sex. Start a monthly meet-up of women to talk about sexuality, relationships, and communication skills. Set aside time to talk to your partner (or partners) about what you like sexually, what you want to try, and what you need as far as communication. Let sex positivity permeate every area of your life so that when the next popular book with a sexual bent comes out, you can proudly read it on the train, on the elliptical, or in line at the store without worrying what people might think of you. The sex positive revolution is here: knowledge is power, and the more sexually empowered and knowledgeable women we have, the more wonderful a place this world will be.

In sexual solidarity,

Shanna Katz

Resources

Sexuality Educators

Annie Sprinkle
www.anniesprinkle.org

Barbara Carrellas
www.urbantantra.org

Betty Dodson and Carlin Ross
www.dodsonandross.com

Carol Queen
www.carolqueen.com

Catherine Toyooka
www.catherinecoaches.com

Charlie Glickman
www.charlieglickman.com

Dr. Jenni Skyler
www.theintimacyinstitute.org

Dr. Petra
www.drpetra.co.uk

Ducky Doolittle
www.duckydoolittle.com

Eve Minax
www.mistressminax.com

Graydancer
www.graydancer.com

Jamye Waxman
www.jamyewaxman.com

Justine Shuey
www.drshuey.com

Julian Wolf
www.julianwolf.net

Lee Harrington
www.passionandsoul.com

Lillith Grey
www.lillithgrey.com

Lolita Wolf
www.leatheryenta.com

Lou Paget
www.loupaget.com

Megan Andelloux
www.ohmegan.com

Midori
www.planetmidori.com

Mollena William
www.mollena.com

Nina Hartley
www.nina.com

Pucker Up — Tristan Taormino
www.puckerup.com

Reid Mihalko
www.reidaboutsex.com

Sarah Sloane
www.sarahsloane.net

Sinclair Sexsmith
www.mrsexsmith.com

Susie Bright
www.susiebright.com

Violet Blue
www.tinynibbles.com

Sexual Health Information Resources

About.com—Sexuality
A clearinghouse of information on all types and facets of sexuality.
sexuality.about.com

American Sexual Health Association
One of the main associations looking into, creating policy around, and doing research on sexual health.
www.ASHAsexualhealth.org

Diva Cup
Reusable menstrual products.
www.divacup.com

It's Your Sex Life
Run by MTV, this website has all sorts of sexuality info, especially about birth control, STIs, consent, and more. Though originally designed for teens/young people, it's good for all ages.
www.itsyoursexlife.com

The Keeper
Reusable menstrual products.
www.keeper.com

MoonCup
Reusable menstrual products.
www.mooncup.co.uk

National HIV/STD Testing Resources
A clearinghouse of information on where you can get HIV and STD testing done locally.
HIVtest.cdc.gov

Our Bodies, Ourselves
The site for the groundbreaking work *Our Bodies, Ourselves*, which delves into women and their sexualities.
www.ourbodiesourselves.org

Planned Parenthood
A pro-choice organization in the United States offering preventive screenings, yearly exams, birth control, STI testing and treatment, and more.
www.PlannedParenthood.org

Scarleteen
A super-informative and accessible website designed for teens but great for all ages.
www.scarleteen.com

Sexuality Information and Education Council of the United States
The main governing body for sexuality education and information in the United States.
www.SIECUS.org

Soft Cup
Reusable menstrual products.
www.softcup.com

Sex Positive or Woman-Owned Toy Stores in the United States and Canada

Ever wander into an "adult" store and feel grossed out or like you were simply not welcome? Never fear! The last two decades have brought us a plethora of sex toy stores run by people who believe in sex positivity, in everyone deserving education on sexuality, and in providing items that are safe for use with different bodies. Many of these stores are also owned and operated by women, ensuring that women and couples (and everyone else who's a little shy or nervous) have a safe place to go to buy items and have their questions accurately answered.

Arizona

Glendale, Northsight, Scottsdale, Tempe, Tolleson, and Tucson
Fascinations
www.funlove.com

California

Oakland
Feelmore 510
www.feelmore510.com
Good Vibrations
www.goodvibes.com

Berkeley
Good Vibrations
www.goodvibes.com

San Francisco
Good Vibrations
www.goodvibes.com

Ventura
Kama Sutra Closet
www.kamasutracloset.com

Los Angeles
The Pleasure Chest
www.thepleasurechest.com

Colorado

Arvada, Aurora, Boulder, Cherry Creek, Colorado Springs, and Lakewood
Fascinations
www.funlove.com

Illinois

Chicago
Early to Bed
www.early2bedshop.com
The Pleasure Chest
www.thepleasurechest.com

Maine

Portland
Nomia
www.nomiaboutique.com

Maryland

Baltimore
Sugar
www.sugartheshop.com

Massachusetts

Brookline
Good Vibrations
www.goodvibes.com

Minnesota

Minneapolis
Smitten Kitten
www.smittenkittenonline.com

New Mexico

Albuquerque
Self Serve
www.selfservetoys.com

New York

New York City
Babeland
www.babeland.com

The Pleasure Chest
www.thepleasurechest.com

Purple Passion
www.purplepassion.com

Oregon

Portland
She Bop
www.sheboptheshop.com

Pennsylvania

Philadelphia
Passional
www.passionalboutique.com

The Velvet Lily
www.thevelvetlily.com

Texas

Austin
Forbidden Fruit
www.forbiddenfruit.com

Washington

Seattle
Babeland
www.babeland.com

Wisconsin

Madison
A Woman's Touch
www.sexualityresources.com

Milwaukee
The Tool Shed
www.toolshedtoys.com

Canada

Toronto
Come As You Are
www.comeasyouare.com

Good for Her
www.goodforher.com

British Columbia
Womyn's Ware
www.womynsware.com

Ottawa

Venus Envy
www.venusenvy.ca

Online Only

Grand Opening!
www.grandopening.com

Stockroom.com
www.stockroom.com

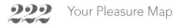

Body-Friendly Sex-Toy Manufacturers

Here's a list of manufacturers committed to making phthalate-free sex toys that are safe for you and your partner to use on your bodies. Some sell directly through their website, and others distribute their products at sex positive and women-owned sex toy stores.

Agreeable Agony — Kinky toys
www.agreeableagony.com

Aneros — Plastic butt toys, prostate toys
www.aneros.com

Aslan Leather — Leather and vegan harnesses, kink toys
www.aslanleather.com

Bad Dragon — Silicone dildos of animals
www.bad-dragon.com

Big Teaze Toys — Plastic vibrators
www.bigteazetoys.com

Crystal Delights — Glass butt toys, dildos, other
www.crystaldelights.com

Fun Factory — Silicone vibrators, dildos, butt toys, Kegel balls, other
www.funfactory.co.uk

Fuze — Silicone butt toys, dildos, other
www.fuzetoys.com

Goldfrau — Ceramic Dildos
www.dildesign.com

Happy Valley — Silicone dildos, butt toys, other
www.happyvalleysilicone.com

Hitachi Magic Wand — Vibrator
www.hitachimagic.com

JeJoue — Silicone vibrators, Kegel balls
www.jejoue.com

Jimmy Jane — Silicone vibrators, massage candles
www.jimmyjane.com

Laid — Silicone dildos, cock rings
www.laid.no

LELO — Silicone vibrators, dildos, butt toys, Kegel balls, sensation play items
www.lelo.com

Minna — Silicone vibrators
www.minnalife.com

NJOY — Stainless steel dildos, butt toys
www.njoytoys.com

NobEssence — Wooden dildos, butt toys
www.nobessence.com

OhMiBod — Plastic iPod-compatible vibrators
www.ohmibod.com

PleasureWorks — Silicone vibrators, dildos, other
www.pleasureworkswholesale.com

Phallix — Glass dildos
www.phallixglass.com

Prysm Creations — Kink toys
www.prysmcreations.com

SpareParts — Harnesses
www.myspare.com

Sportsheets — Harnesses, light bondage items, other
www.sportsheets.com

Square Peg Toys — Silicone dildos, kinky toys, butt toys
www.squarepegtoys.com

Tantus — Silicone dildos, butt toys, vibrators, paddles
www.tantusinc.com

Vergenza — Aluminum dildos
www.inspiredbyvergenza.com

Vixen Creations — Silicone dildos, butt toys, other
www.vixencreations.com

We-Vibe — Silicone vibrators
www.we-vibe.com

Vibratex — Elastomer and TPR vibrators, penis sleeves, butt toys, other
www.vibratex.com

Zeta Paws — Silicone dildos of animals
www.zoofur.com

Body-Friendly, Glycerin-Free Lubricants

Here's a list of companies dedicated to making good-quality lube that's safe for use on all types of bodies. Most of these are paraben-free, and all are lye- and glycerin-free!

Aloe Cadabera — Water based, vegan
www.aloecadabra.com

Blossom Organics — Water based, warming, massage oil
www.blossom-organics.com

Bodyglide by Pjur and Eros — Silicone based
www.pjurusa.com and www.eros-lube .com

Earthly Body — Water based, massage oil, massage candles
www.earthlybody.com

Hathor — Water based, massage oil, vegan
www.hathorbody.com

Maximus — Water based, does have some parabens
www.maximuslube.com

Nature Labs — Water based
www.naturelovinlubricants.com

O'My — Water based, flavored
www.omyonline.com

Pre-Seed — Water based, fertility, contains parabens
www.preseed.com

Sliquid — Water based, silicone based, flavored, all vegan
www.sliquid.com

Uberlube — Silicone based
www.uberlube.com

Yes — Water based, massage oil/oil based, vegan
www.yesyesyes.org

Top-Notch Pornography Sites and Companies

Sites

AbbyWinters.com
theArtOfTheBlowJob.com
BeautifulAgony.com
BurningAngel.com
CrashPadSeries.com
ForTheGirls.com
GoodDykePorn.com
HotMoviesForHer.com
IndiePornRevolution.com
QueerPorn.TV

Companies

C.Batts Fly Productions
Comstock Films
Feelmore Ent.
Femme Productions
Filly Films
Girl Candy Films
Good Releasing
Hard Candy Productions
Heart Core Productions
JoyBear Pictures
Juicy Pink Box
Julie Simone Productions
Lust Films
Mayhem Multimedia
Petra Joy
Pink and White Productions
Reel Queer Productions
Sweetheart Video
Sweet Sinners Video
Trouble Films
Vivid-Ed Series

Index

A

Allergic reactions
  condoms, 211
  lubricants, 124
  sex toys, 92
Anal beads, 147–148
Analingus. *See* Oral
  sex
Anal numbing
  products, 132
Anal plugs, 149–150
Anal sex, 129–151
  cautions, 130
  cleanliness, 134–136,
    144, 150
  communication with
    partner about, 133,
    136–139
  condom use, 135–
    136, 142
  dildo use, 144–146,
    150–151
  ending, 142–144
  foreplay before,
    140–141
  lubrication for, 134,
    145, 147, 151
  numbing products,
    132
  orgasm before, 133
  orgasm during,
    142–143

pain during, 129–130,
    132
  relaxation strategies,
    131–134
  safer sex precautions,
    135–136, 142, 147,
    150–151
  sex toy use, 104, 118,
    144, 146–151
  slow and steady
    method, 140–142
Anal stimulation, 75,
    134, 143
Anatomy, of vulva,
    153–155
Ankles, 47
Armpits, 48

B

Bars, as date location,
    16, 18
BDSM (bondage and
  discipline, sadism,
  and masochism),
  170. *See also* Kinky
  sex
Beads
  anal, 147–148
  for Kegel muscle
    strengthening,
    104–105

Bend Over Boyfriend,
    146
Ben Wa Balls, 104
Best Women's Erotica,
    79
Bets, as dating activity,
    8
Blindfolds, 73, 92, 98
Blood pressure, 66,
    67, 70
"Blue balls," 68
Bondage, 188–196
  cuffs, 188–189,
    191–193
  handcuff caution,
    188–189
  ropes, 194–196
  ties or scarves, 92,
    141, 189–191
Books, 78–81
Bottoming, 174–176
Boy shorts, 36
Bras, 37
Breaking the ice,
    201–202
Breasts
  nipple stimulation, 44
  before orgasm, 66
BurningAngel.com, 83
Bustiers, 37
Butt beads, 147–148
Butt plugs, 149–150

Acknowledgments

It goes without saying that my partner, Leo, has been an incredible support in the creation of this book, from responding when I called out for another synonym for getting it on, to validating me for locking myself in to write for hours on end. Thank you, oh stud muffin of mine, for being such an amazing partner in all things, all the time.

All three kitties (Kinsey, Kali, and Jasper) were there every step of the way, keeping my lap warm, closing my laptop when I had been on it too long, and providing comic, furry relief at needed times.

My family never once questioned my drive to become a professional pervert, so to my mother, Hedy, and sister, Risa, thank you for your unwavering encouragement.

A big thanks to my editor at Amorata Press, Katherine, who handled my sense of humor, random inquiries, and sometimes annoying attention to semantics with grace and courtesy ... even when I was being overly nitpicky.

Lastly, a huge thank you to all of the amazing sex-positive toy stores, sex toy companies, and educators who have worked tirelessly for years, and continue to work hard every day, to create a safe space for sexual exploration for people of all identities. Whether it is answering questions, providing access to information and/or sex accessories, or creating products that are not only body friendly but designed with human pleasure in mind, it is the work of these individuals, companies, and organizations that moves the field of sexuality forward, each and every day. I have done my best to list many of them here, but hopefully these lists continue to grow and grow until everyone has access to fun, relevant, and positive information and support around sexuality.

About the Author

Shanna Katz, M.Ed, ACS, is a queer, kinky, board-certified sexologist, sexuality educator, and author. From topics like relationship communication skills to non-monogamy, and oral sex to how sexuality and dis/ability intersect, she talks, writes, and teaches about the huge spectrum of sexuality, both from personal and from professional perspectives. She's given presentations at Brown University, the University of Arizona, SUNY-Purchase, University of Pennsylvania, Princeton, and Colorado College, and facilitated the American Medical Student Association's Sexual Health Scholars Program. She also offers workshops at sex-toy stores, LGBT centers, women's groups, and kink conferences around the country.

Shanna is using her Master's of Sexuality Education to provide accessible, open-source sex education to people around the world as she works toward her PhD in Social Work. Shanna's first two books are *Oral Sex That'll Blow Her Mind: An Illustrated Guide to Giving Her Amazing Orgasms* and *Lesbian Sex Positions: 100 Passionate Positions from Intimate and Sensual to Wild and Naughty*, and her erotica has been published in *Wetter, Love Notes, The Lust Chronicles*, and other anthologies. Her writing can be found in *Out Front Colorado*, the *Fearless Press*, GoodVibes.com, Feministing.com, and in many more places both online and in print. Shanna lives with her partner and their three kitties in Colorado. For more info, please visit www.ShannaKatz .com, friend her on Facebook, or follow her @Shanna_Katz.

Made in United States
Orlando, FL
05 January 2023

28278650R00135